Decoding Bipolar Disorder: Practical Treatment and Management

by

Trisha Suppes, MD, PhD
J. Sloan Manning, MD
Paul E. Keck, Jr., MD

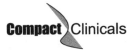

Compact Clinicals

This book is prepared and presented as a service to the medical community by Compact Clinics, with support from AstraZeneca Pharmaceuticals LP. The information provided reflects the published literature as well as the knowledge, experience, and personal opinions of the authors, Trisha Suppes, MD, PhD; J. Sloan Manning, MD; and Paul E. Keck, Jr. MD and does not reflect recommendations by AstraZeneca.

This book is not intended to replace or to be used as a substitute for the complete prescribing information prepared for each drug by its respective manufacturer. To be certain that you have the most current data, always consult the manufacturer's current prescribing information before prescribing or administering any products described in this publication.

Published by:
Compact Clinics
7205 N.W. Waukomis, Kansas City, MO 64151
816-587-0044

Medical Writing/Editing/Concept Development:
Kathi L. Whitman, In Credible English, Kansas City, MO

Medical Editing: Adi R. Ferrara, Seattle, WA

Library of Congress Cataloging-in-Publication Data

Suppes, Trisha
Decoding bipolar disorder : practical treatment and management / by
    Trisha Suppes, J. Sloan Manning, Paul E. Keck Jr.
        p.   ; cm.
    Includes bibliographical references.
    ISBN 13-978-1-887537-29-2
    ISBN 1-887537-29-5
    1. Manic-depressive illness. I. Manning, J. Sloan (James Sloan),
1957-   . II. Keck, Paul E. III. Title.
    [DNLM: 1. Bipolar Disorder–diagnosis. 2. Bipolar Disorder–
    therapy. WM 207 S959d 2007]
    RC516.D4344 2007
    616.89'5--dc22

                                                        2006032429

                Printed in the United States of America
                10   9   8   7   6   5   4   3   2   1

Table of Contents

Dedications

To Deborah for her wonderful support
and problem solving skills
(Trisha Suppes)

To my wife, Jana, and sons,
Joshua and Jonathan – all touched by the
gifts and pain of bipolar illness
(Sloan Manning)

For Tim and Jason, and
the joy they have brought to my life
(Paul Keck)

Foreword

Decoding bipolar disorder remains a diagnostic and treatment challenge for all health practitioners — psychiatrist and primary care physician alike.

This illness presents itself in a variety of different forms, requires flexible and ever-changing treatment strategies, and may follow an unpredictable course. Making a definitive diagnosis is crucial. Developing a medication treatment plan involves balancing efficacy, tolerability, and safety. Improving treatment compliance and outcomes necessitates consistent patient monitoring as well as patient education into the nature of the disorder and the role of medication treatment. Each individual's response is unique. Effective, long-term management depends on a comprehensive, collaborative health care approach that integrates primary care and mental health services using a chronic care model.

> *Current DSM-IV(TR) criteria requires occurrence of a defined hypomanic or manic episode. This requirement may delay proper diagnosis and treatment of the early-onset, recurrent bipolar depressions that often herald the onset of illness and precede hypomania and mania.*

Bipolar disorder is neither rare nor merely manic illness. Depression creates a significant burden and is the phase of illness that most often presents to clinicians. Often symptoms of mania and depression are concurrent (mixed) with the patient's particular symptom mixture significantly influencing both symptomatic presentation and treatment strategy.

Beyond the diagnostic challenges of identifying bipolar illness when patients present as depressed, **the iatrogenic impacts of misdiagnosis and antidepressant monotherapy may significantly worsen bipolar disorder course** and severely hamper the effectiveness of future treatments for many patients. Thus, there is a strong need for:

- Making unipolar major depression a diagnosis of exclusion.
- Helping clinicians become better diagnosticians, who eschew potentially harmful treatment strategies when any significant diagnostic uncertainty exists.
- **Not** viewing mental illness as fundamentally different from general medical conditions. The proper assessment and treatment of mental health conditions follows the same standard clinical paradigm as other illnesses, such as diabetes or hypertension.

In the best models of care, there is a longitudinal involvement with the patient and thus, the course of the illness. **Bipolar illness has a longitudinal trajectory that requires attention to risk factors, prodromal and syndromal manifestations, and health consequences.** At every point of interaction with patients, the clinician needs an accurate portrayal of what the illness is and where it comes from and where it's going.

Psychiatrists and primary care practitioners may find it useful to review the life cycle, biopsychosocial nature, and longitudinal course of bipolar illness as with other chronic illnesses. With hypertension, for example, there are inherited vulnerabilities, there is an interplay of psychosocial and lifestyle components, and there are outcomes that, in retrospect, represent lost opportunities for earlier diagnosis as well as secondary or tertiary prevention strategies. Primary care physicians see people regularly in their practices with congestive cardiomyopathies resulting from hypertension before a hypertension diagnosis has been made. When this happens, clinicians typically ask themselves, "Could this have been prevented or the effects minimized?"

And so it is with bipolar disorder. There are inherited vulnerabilities, family history "red flags," early onset clues linked to temperament and prodromal (usually depressive) fluctuations in mood, and psychosocial stressors that can precipitate manic or depressive episodes. There are also the outcomes that perhaps could have been avoided. There are marriages lost, jobs lost, substance abuse, people who become (through misdiagnosis or mismanagement) almost impossible to treat, suicides — all the outcomes that provoke the question, "What could have been done differently 10 years ago to help prevent some of these outcomes?"

Key factors for clinicians "decoding" the diagnostic and treatment issues surrounding bipolar disorder include the illness':

- **Strong heritability** — The primary care practitioner may have more access to family history.

- **Longitudinal trajectory** — A lifespan perspective of health care helps clinicians appreciate the roots of the illness in early age temperament, especially when multi-generational families are seen in a practice.

  > *Anticipating the possibility of bipolar illness when encountering patients with early onset and chronic/recurrent depressive illness is critical.*

- **Medical comorbidity** — Primary care practitioners' inherent comprehensive approach to treatment can be vital in both diagnosis and management of patients suffering from bipolar illness and other associated medical conditions. Psychiatrists need to be comfortable recognizing and treating or "triaging" comorbid medical disorders.

- **Need for a sensitive approach to treatment** — The presence of an existing therapeutic alliance with a primary provider may improve communication and add a helpful voice in treatment, particularly regarding the existential qualities of the illness that are essential to successful management.

- **Challenges for treatment adherence** — Patients being treated for bipolar disorder need close monitoring to ensure treatment compliance and ongoing management. Psychiatrists play a vital role in the collaborative treatment process; primary care physicians may "close the loop" due to the more comprehensive nature of their relationships with their patients.

> *Primary care physicians need to remain engaged in the bipolar treatment process because they can contribute a great deal to effective comprehensive management of this illness.*

Clinicians will make choices about referral, consultation, and/or collaboration depending on the clinical scenario. Collaborative care may offer everyone involved — patient, primary care clinician, and psychiatrist — a better chance to "decode" bipolar illness.

Chapter 1: About Bipolar Disorder

For those with bipolar disorder, as well as for their families and friends, life is an unpredictable and debilitating series of emotional highs and lows. Often referred to in the past as manic-depression, bipolar disorder represents a biological condition characterized by mood swings that are often severe and even life-threatening. After any manic episode, mild or severe, people with bipolar disorder may experience depression or a symptom-free phase (euthymia). Eventually, in most untreated individuals, a depressive episode ensues.

Depression is the most common expression of the illness and responsible for most of the morbidity and mortality (25–55 percent suicide incidence rate) associated with the illness.[1]

Complicating this picture further are the diagnostic challenges inherent in the management of the disorder — over 30 percent of patients with bipolar illness are incorrectly diagnosed with unipolar depression and nearly another 50 percent with some other disorder.[2] Inappropriate treatment or under-treatment can exacerbate symptoms, often increasing "switches to mania or accelerating the cycle of mood swings."[3]

Those with untreated bipolar disorder are typically unstable, experiencing uncomfortable and unpredictable mood states as well as changes in energy, sleep, and behavior. Even when treated, medications may have to be adjusted as patients face new episodes or breakthrough symptoms. However, with effective medication treatment, many patients experience a reduction or remission in symptoms.

SECTION A: INTRODUCTION TO BIPOLAR DISORDER – THE ILLNESS

How Bipolar Disorder Impacts Patients' Lives

Current research indicates a need to reconceptualize bipolar illness as a highly recurrent, extremely pleomorphic, and potentially lethal medical disorder. The time frame from when a patient's symptoms first meet DSM criteria to initial treatment averages a decade, making earlier diagnosis and intervention critical.[1]

Those with bipolar disorder typically find that their quality of life and ability to function changes, even with adequate treatment and symptom remission.[4-7] Symptom patterns vary depending on whether the person is experiencing depressive, manic, hypomanic, or mixed episodes. Early recognition of these episodes as part of the overall spectrum of the disorder is key to early diagnosis and effective treatment.

When symptoms persist untreated, those with bipolar disorder may face a high risk for unpredictable and often dangerous behavior as well as self-injury and suicide. In addition, they are at risk when they fail to take medications as prescribed or experience limited response to treatment.[8, 9]

Specific Impacts of Depression

Many patients who may ultimately be diagnosed with bipolar illness initially present only with depressive symptoms, not recognizing manic or hypomanic periods. The differential diagnosis of unipolar (major depression only) from bipolar is critical for all patients presenting with depression (see chapter 7 for more detail). Key "red flags" that a patient presenting with depression may suffer from bipolar depression rather than unipolar depression have to do with the person having:

- A family history of mood disorders
- A psychohistory of "energized" or "irritable" depression
- More severe episodes

- Inadequate response to previous treatment for depression
- An early age of onset for depressive symptoms

Depressed people often have trouble concentrating, remembering, and making decisions. They may be unable to concentrate on a television program or book, decide what to wear, or whether to renew a subscription, feeling that these decisions are overwhelming or exhausting. Persons with depression report very low self-esteem,

Typical Depression Symptoms
Loss of interest/pleasure in activities once enjoyed (including sex)
Changes in appetite/weight
Decreased energy, concentration, memory
Increased feelings of hopelessness, pessimism, guilt, worthlessness, anxiety, helplessness
Fatigue, irritability, restlessness
Chronic pain (not caused by physical illness or injury)
Suicidal thoughts and/or attempts

and often dwell on their negative qualities, failings, or losses. They also report feelings of hopelessness: a belief that nothing will ever improve; exaggerated pessimism. For someone with bipolar depression, these symptoms may have some element of agitation or animation mixed in with the sad, dejected mannerisms.

Specific Impacts of Hypomania

Hypomania is an observable change from usual function that is not as severe as mania, but still constitutes an unstable mood state. Hypomania may be a dark, disruptive kind of experience; patients tend to be more prone to making impulsive decisions, which can have lasting consequences.

Hypomania presents unusual diagnostic challenges, especially since the symptom presentation may be more global in nature than specific DSM criteria for a syndromal "episode" might indicate. Individuals experiencing hypomania may feel great and even associate their symptoms with optimal functioning and enhanced productivity. However,

INTRODUCTION

PRESENTATION

CLINICAL PROCESS

PHARMACOTHERAPY

RESOURCES

this period is often one of restless, driven, irritable mood that can be very unpleasant for the patient and others. Those with hypomania can feel sad as well as elevated and even irritable — within a very short span of time. Often these symptoms go unreported to clinicians because patients perceive them as somewhat positive and beneficial. Even when family and friends learn to recognize the mood swings as possible bipolar disorder, the person may deny that anything is wrong. Family members may note that the patient is active during periods where one would expect otherwise. For example, someone who experiences a mixture of hypomanic and depressive symptoms (depressive mixed state) might complete intensive coursework to earn their MBA during a period when family members saw the same person as being very depressed.

Without proper treatment, however, hypomania can lead to more severe mania or herald a period of ongoing mood instability. That same patient who completed the MBA might have gone six months without a "syndromal" hypomanic episode, but during a routine visit, laughs and jokes with the primary care physician one minute and talks about suicidal thoughts the next.

Specific Impacts of Mania

Mania is energy; its energetic qualities are severely dysfunctional, intense, and troubling to the patient and others.

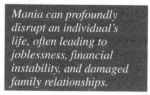

Mania can profoundly disrupt an individual's life, often leading to joblessness, financial instability, and damaged family relationships.

Typically, those experiencing a manic episode find they sleep less or not at all due to a disruption in their circadian rhythms. Despite this, they sustain high energy levels (e.g., a person in a full manic episode may feel little or no need for sleep, exercise several hours daily, and have "boundless" energy for new projects). However, this energy may not be focused in a productive fashion, and the patient may go for many days without sleeping. In fact, patients in the 19th century (prior to medication treatment) would sometimes die from manic episodes due to lack of sleep and neglecting to eat or drink water.

Classic mania may be associated with being distinctly self-confident (grandiosity) and behavior that family and friends recognize as atypical for the individual, such as: spending sprees, promiscuity, alcohol or drug abuse, or other impulsive, potentially risky behavior. Patients with bipolar disorder may neither recognize their symptoms nor, as mania worsens, the consequences of their risky behavior because of the confusion and loss of contact with reality that occurs when the disorder remains untreated.

Specific Impacts of Mixed Episodes

Many patients experience a mix of symptoms, with depressive symptoms either occurring simultaneously or within a short time of hypomanic or manic symptoms — a presentation considered a mixed form of mania. For example, a patient could be very irritable with a depressed mood and also feel very energized and make impulsive decisions. Patients may also experience mixed symptoms without meeting full criteria for either mania or depression.

Such mixtures do not have to be full, concurrent episodes of mania and major depression.[10] Hypomania and mania can contain significant, but sub-syndromal, depressive symptoms. These manifestations are termed, "dysphoric." Conversely, depression can be tinged with sub-syndromal levels of manic symptoms, and the patient can appear agitated or excited and impulsive.

Symptoms of a mixed bipolar state often also include trouble sleeping, significant change in appetite, refractory anxiety (even panic states), psychosis, and suicidal thinking.

Mixed episodes are often severe and impair daily functioning in social interactions, occupational activity, and intimate relationships. A mixed episode can last from one week to several months, generally followed by a depressive episode. Women are more prone to mixed episodes.

INTRODUCTION

PRESENTATION

CLINICAL PROCESS

PHARMACOTHERAPY

RESOURCES

In teenagers, mixed episodes occur most frequently among those who have experienced major depression. In children, this may be the primary presentation.

Bipolar Disorder and Primary Care

Because a significant percent of the care of psychiatric patients is done in the primary care setting, bipolar disorder has a prevalent and important place in primary care practice.[11]

Although primary care physicians welcomed serotonin reuptake inhibitors in the 1990s as safe, broad-spectrum agents for diverse patients encountered in daily practice, emerging data indicates a need to shift from emphasizing antidepressants to early identification of the bipolar diathesis.[12] Key concepts related to this shift include:

> *Regardless of ultimate decisions regarding treatment management, primary care remains the first line of defense in recognizing and treating bipolar disorder. This is because depression, the most common expression of the illness, presents principally to the primary care sector.*

1. **Understanding that bipolar disorder is neither rare nor merely manic illness** — Although specifically identified by the presence or history of mania or hypomania, it is depression that creates the greatest burden of illness and is the phase of illness that most often presents to clinicians.[13, 14]

2. **Symptoms of depression, hypomania, and mania are often concurrent (mixed)** — The particular mixture of mania and depression is common, variable, and often unrecognized or confused with agitated depression or refractory anxiety states. In fact, one large cohort study of well-characterized patients with bipolar disorder found an increased probability for both sexes to experience mixed symptoms when hypomanic.[15] Mixed states typically last longer and recur more often with an elevated risk for suicide.

3. **Current DSM-IV(TR) criteria emphasis may delay proper diagnosis of early onset bipolar disorder** — Because DSM-IV(TR) calls for a hypomanic or manic episode prior to an official bipolar diagnosis, there can be a resulting delay in proper diagnosis and treatment of early onset illness.[10] The recurrent depressions that often herald bipolar onset can precede hypomania and mania, making anticipation of a diagnosis an important consideration.

4. **Unipolar major depression should be approached as a diagnosis of exclusion** — Patients with bipolar II disorder are frequently misdiagnosed with unipolar depression because both patient and clinician struggle to recognize hypomanic periods, perhaps because of the expectation that hypomania is predominately euphoric. It is extremely common for patients with symptoms of hypomania, especially women, to actually have mixed hypomania — a condition characterized as "energized depression."[15]

5. **Clinicians must avoid potentially harmful treatment strategies whenever diagnostic uncertainty exists** — In patients with bipolar illness, antidepressant monotherapy has been linked to increased mood cycling or lack of response.[15]

The Course of Bipolar Illness

The longitudinal course of bipolar illness is highly unpredictable. What the disorder looks like today in any given individual may be quite different than how it presents five years in the future. Key to diagnosis and management for primary care clinicians is to look for elements that help rule out bipolar disorder. For example, a patient that presents with symptoms that "look" like mania but has no family history of mood disorders might either be:

• Withholding information about family history due to perceived stigma

• Unaware of family psychiatric history
• Suffering from some other disorder with symptoms somewhat like bipolar disorder

Looking at the longitudinal course of bipolar disorder is much the same as for non-psychiatric conditions. For example, note the relationship of course between type II diabetes and bipolar disorder in figure 1.1 on the next page in terms of inherited vulnerabilities and psychosocial/lifestyle components as well as lost opportunities for earlier diagnosis.

One of the most challenging features of bipolar disorder is that patients' experiences of the illness can vary tremendously, with some patients suffering depression followed by hypomania, and others mania followed by depression. Some move quickly from episode to episode, with virtually no period of mood stability (euthymia) in between significant ups and downs. Others may be relatively stable between discrete episodes of mania or depression for longer periods.

Treatment challenges include:

• **Conceptualizing the bipolar spectrum** — Bipolar disorder, in general, is a dimensional illness with a full spectrum of mood episodes.[16]

• **Realizing that the dominant symptomatic course of bipolar illness may be depressive rather than manic/hypomanic** — Breakthrough depression typically poses greater problems for long-term treatment than mania.[1]

These mood manifestations may not meet criteria for any of the specific DSM-IV(TR) bipolar diagnoses — BD-I, BD-II, or BD-NOS (see pages 123 through 125 for definitions/criteria for each). For example, some see "bipolarity" as a dimensional illness continuous from BD-I through entities not currently categorized by DSM-IV(TR) (e.g., borderline bipolar, soft bipolar, and affective temperaments, such as

Figure 1.1 Longitudinal Course Comparison

Impacting Elements	Type II Diabetes Mellitus	Bipolar Disorder
Pedigree (Family History)	• Inherited vulnerability	• Inherited vulnerability • Predisposing temperamental factors (e.g., mood lability)
Lifestyle/ Environmental Contributions	• Sedentary • Obese	• Poor sleep hygiene • Substance use (alcohol, stimulants) • Trauma, abuse (especially as children or adolescents)
Sub-syndromal Heralds	• Insulin resistance • Hypertension • Decreased HDL (high-density lipoprotein)	• Recurrent brief depressions, often in childhood or adolescence, especially mixed with irritability and acting out
Syndromal Indicators Easily Overlooked	• Postprandial hyperglycemia • Nocturia	• Major depression with hypomanic features (depressive mixed states) or with brief hypomanic-like periods (BD-NOS)
Syndromal Illness	• Abnormal fasting glucose	• Hypomania or mania
Outcomes that Represent Lost Opportunities for Earlier Diagnosis	• Neuropathy • Nephropathy • Coronary artery disease	• Marital or economic disruption • Treatment resistance • Suicide

INTRODUCTION

PRESENTATION

CLINICAL PROCESS

PHARMACOTHERAPY

RESOURCES

> *Familiarity with these dimensional aspects of bipolar disorder, especially temperament, can be invaluable for effective treatment, but it takes time and being engaged with the patient.*

hyperthymic, cyclothymic, dysthymic, irritable) and in-between disorders (e.g., bipolar III).[17–19] Further research is needed to determine the link between this interface of symptoms and "temperament" and subsequent implications for illness course and treatment.

- **Defining each patient's individual characteristic pattern at any phase of the illness** — Primary care clinicians, who often have repetitive, longitudinal contact with bipolar patients for various health care issues, are in a position to help identify and track such patterns. They may also have established therapeutic relationships that would help patients better understand those patterns through effective psychoeducation programs.

- **Managing the problems of treatment resistance in bipolar disorder** — The Stanley Foundation Bipolar Network study found over 40 percent of patients remained intermittently ill despite treatment.[1]

- **Managing suicide risk** — Clinicians need to consider suicide risk for patients with bipolar disorder and mitigate that risk, especially among those with mixed episodes (dysphoric mania).[15]

Because both bipolar illness diagnosis and treatment is a longitudinal process, patients and their health care providers need to establish and cultivate a working therapeutic alliance. In such an alliance, both patient and provider learn to become "experts" in the patient's illness. Both must recognize individual symptom expressions, including reproducible symptom patterns as well as psychosocial context and environmental factors that can impact the course of the illness.

Environmental Factors that Influence Bipolar Illness Course

A number of environmental factors influence the course of bipolar illness from diagnosis to treatment to maintenance to prognosis. These include practical/lifestyle issues, ethnicity issues and utilization of services, substance abuse comorbidity, number of untreated episodes, and major life stressors.

> *Although not an "environmental factor" per se, head injury can contribute to onset of bipolar illness as well as to a mood "switch" for those already experiencing symptoms.*

Practical/Lifestyle Issues

For many people, the stigma of having been diagnosed with bipolar disorder can make it very difficult to obtain health and life insurance benefits or to gain employment or advance one's career. Additionally, those with bipolar disorder are less likely to be successful in jobs that require frequent shift changes or travel between time zones. Changes in sleep-wake cycles that occur with sleep deprivation or international travel can precipitate or exacerbate manic, hypomanic, or mixed episodes.[10]

Because of the side effects of some bipolar medications (drowsiness), operating heavy machinery, doing high-rise construction work, or driving a commercial vehicle could be very problematic.

Ethnicity and Utilization of Services

A number of studies indicate that ethnic minorities experience a different course of treatment and utilization of services than Caucasians. Examples include being more likely to be involuntarily committed to hospitals, attempt suicide, have shorter lengths of stay when hospitalized (for those who are non-psychotic), or be observed less closely.[20–24]

In a 2005 study that specifically looked at patients with bipolar disorder, minorities were more often involuntarily committed as inpatients. This phenomenon was present

INTRODUCTION

PRESENTATION

CLINICAL PROCESS

PHARMACOTHERAPY

RESOURCES

even after adjusting for age, gender, current substance use disorder, and psychosis.[25]

Treatment for Asian patients can be challenging as this group tends to have certain sensitivities and side effects with various pharmacotherapies not typically experienced by other ethnic minorities or Caucasians.[26–32]

> As very few studies exist on racial/ethnic differences, this area represents a key gap in our current knowledge base.

Substance Abuse Comorbidity

There is a high risk for adolescents and young adult patients, especially those who have not been diagnosed properly for bipolar illness, to acquire severe liabilities in terms of comorbid alcohol and substance abuse.[1] In addition, there is an increased risk of dependence among women with bipolar illness.[1]

Untreated Episodes

The more untreated episodes (both manic and depressive in nature) a person suffers, the less favorable the prognosis for general and combination treatment.[1]

Major Life Stressors

Stressful events can precipitate relapse.[33] Alternately, life events associated with positive goals can increase manic symptoms.[34]

The Stanley Foundation Bipolar Network study of 632 patients with bipolar disorder found the following stressors associated with suicide attempts:[1]

- **Course of illness** — Increased severity of mania, more time ill, and early onset
- **Comorbidities** — Anxiety, eating disorders, Axis II disorders
- **Occupational, financial, and health care adversities** — Problems with health insurance and access to heath care

- **Social Support Systems** — Death of important other, lack of a confidant
- **Genetics** — Family history of suicide and substance abuse

The Stanley Foundation study also found that these stressors, when experienced early in the patient's life, appeared to be precursors of ongoing accumulation of stressors, lack of social support, and inadequate access to medical care.[1]

Effective communication between patients with bipolar disorder and primary care clinicians often requires becoming a "student" of the patient and creating an atmosphere of empathetic openness. This approach invites the patient to provide details essential for optimal treatment and stabilization. In the role of educator and wise counsel, the clinician can offer information and honest messages about the illness and obstacles to recovery.

References for Chapter 1

1. Post RM, Leverich GS, Altshuler LL, et al. An overview of recent findings of the Stanley Foundation Bipolar Network (Part I). *Bipolar Disorders.* 2003;5:310–19.

2. Hirschfeld RM. The Mood Disorder Questionnaire: a simple, patient-rated screening instrument for bipolar disorder. *Prim Care Companion J Clin Psychiatry.* 2002;4(1):9–11.

3. Goodwin FK, Jamison KR. *Manic-Depressive Illness;* 1990. New York: Oxford University Press.

4. Goldberg JF, Harrow M, Grossman LS. Course and outcome in bipolar affective disorder: a longitudinal follow-up study. *Am J Psychiatry.* 1995;152(3):379–84.

5. Gitlin MJ, Swendsen J, Heller TL, et al. Relapse and impairment in bipolar disorder. *Am J Psychiatry.* 1995;152:1635–40.

6. Coryell W, Scheftner W, Keller M, et al. The enduring psychosocial consequences of mania and depression. *Am J Psychiatry.* 1993;150:720–7.

7. Tohen M, Hennen J, Zarate CM Jr, et al. Two-year syndromal and functional recovery in 219 cases of first-episode major affective disorder with psychotic features. *Am J Psychiatry.* 2000;157(2):220–8.

8. Dilsaver SC, Chen YW, Swann AC, et al. Suicidality in patients with pure and depressive mania. *Am J Psychiatry.* 1994;151:1312–15.

9. Strakowski SM, McElroy SL, Keck PE Jr, et al. Suicidality among patients with mixed and manic bipolar disorder. *Am J Psychiatry*. 1996;153:674–6.

10. American Psychiatric Association, American Psychiatric Association Task Force on DSM-IV. *Diagnostic and statistical manual of mental disorders: DSM-IV-TR*. Washington, DC: American Psychiatric Association; 2000.

11. Norquist GS, Regier DA. The epidemiology of psychiatric disorders and the defacto mental health care system. *Annu. Rev. Med.* 1996;47:473–9.

12. Manning JS, Ahmed S, McGuire HC, et al., Mood disorders in family practice: beyond unipolarity to bipolarity. *Prim Care Companion J Clin Psychiatry*. 2004;6(5):222–3.

13. Manning JS. Burden of illness in bipolar depression. *Prim Care Companion J Clin Psychiatry*. 2005;7(6):259–67.

14. Judd LL, Akiskal HS, Schettler PJ, et al. Psychosocial disability in the course of bipolar I and II disorders: a prospective, comparative, longitudinal study. *Arch Gen Pschiatry*. 2005 Dec;62(12):1322–30.

15. Suppes T, Mintz J, McElroy SL, et al. Mixed hypomania in 908 patients with bipolar disorder evaluated prospectively in the Stanley Foundation Bipolar Treatment Network: a sex-specific phenomenon. *Arch Gen Psychiatry*. 2005 Oct;62:1089–96.

16. Judd LL, Akiskal HS. The prevalence and disability of bipolar spectrum disorders in the US population: re-analysis of the ECA database taking into account subthreshold cases. *J Affect Disord*. 2003 Jan;73(1-2):123–31.

17. Cassano GB, Frank E, Miniati M, et al. Conceptual underpinnings and empirical support for the mood spectrum. *Psychiatr Clin North Am*. 2002;25(4):699–712.

18. Angst J. The emerging epidemiology of hypomania and bipolar II disorder. *J Affect Disord*. 1998;50(2-3):143–51.

19. Akiskal HS, Pinto O. The evolving bipolar spectrum. Prototypes I, II, III, and IV. *Psychiatr Clin North Am*. 1999;22(3):517–34, vii.Review.

20. Davies S, Thornicroft G, Leese M, et al. Ethnic differences in risk of compulsory psychiatric admission among representative cases of psychosis in London. *BMJ*. 1996 Mar;312(7030):533–7.

21. Thomas CS, Stone K, Osborn M, et al. Psychiatric morbidity and compulsory admission among UK-born Europeans, Afro-Caribbeans and Asians in central Manchester. *Br J Psychiatry*. 1993 Jul;163:91–9.

22. Commander MJ, O'Dell SM, Surtees PG, et al. Characteristics of patients and patterns of psychiatric service use in ethnic minorities. *Int J Soc Psychiatry*. 2003 Sep;49(3):216–24.

23. Kupfer DJ, Frank E, Grochocinski VJ, et al. African-American participants in a bipolar disorder registry: clinical and treatment characteristics. *Bipolar Disord*. 2005 Feb;7(1):82–8.

24. Chung H, Mahler JC, Kakuma T. Racial differences in treatment of psychiatric inpatients. *Psychiatr Serv*. 1995 Jun;46(6):586–91.

25. Kilbourne AM, Bauer MS, Pincus H, et al. Veterans Administration (VA) Cooperative Study #430 Team. Clinical, psychosocial, and treatment differences in minority patients with bipolar disorder. *Bipolar Disord*. 2005 Feb;7(1):89–97.

26. Rudorfer MV, Lane EA, Chang WH, et al. Desipramine pharmacokinetics in Chinese and Caucasian volunteers. *Br J Clin Pharmacol*. 1984 Apr;17(4):433–40.

27. Kumana CR, Lauder IJ, Chan M, et al. Differences in diazepam pharmacokinetics in Chinese and white Caucasians--relation to body lipid stores. *Eur J Clin Pharmacol*. 1987;32(2):211–5.

28. Potkin SG, Shen Y, Pardes H, et al. Haloperidol concentrations elevated in Chinese patients. *Psychiatry Res*. 1984 Jun;12(2):167–72.

29. Lane HY, Chiu WC, Chou JC, et al. Risperidone in acutely exacerbated schizophrenia: dosing strategies and plasma levels. *International Journal of Clinical Pharmacology & Therapeutics*. 2000;38(10):482–5.

30. Rosenblat R. Tang SW. Do Oriental psychiatric patients receive different dosages of psychotropic medication when compared with occidentals. *Canadian Journal of Psychiatry — Revue Canadienne de Psychiatrie*. 1987;32(2):211–5.

31. Lin KM, Smith MW, Ortiz V. Culture and psychopharmacology. *Psychiatric Clinics of North America*. 2001;24(3):523–38.

32. Zhou HH, Shay SD, Wood AJ. Contribution of differences in plasma binding of propranolol to ethnic differences in sensitivity. Comparison between Chinese and Caucasians. *Chinese Medical Journal*. 1993;106(12):898–902.

33. Hunt N, Bruce-Jones W, Silverstone T. Life events and relapse in bipolar affective disorder. *J Affect Disord*. 1992;25(1):13–20.

34. Johnson SL, Sandrow D, Meyer B, et al. Increases in manic symptoms after life events involving goal attainment. *J Abnorm Psychol*. 2000;109(4):721–7.

INTRODUCTION

PRESENTATION

CLINICAL PROCESS

PHARMACOTHERAPY

RESOURCES

Chapter 2: Etiology

Bipolar disorder is a mood disorder that appears to be caused by a dysregulation in brain chemistry, which can be exacerbated by genetic factors and "triggered" by environmental situations or events, such as early childhood abuse or major disruptions in sleep/wake cycles.

In recent decades, we've come to understand that bipolar disorder typically stems from instability and malfunction in brain activity, not from environmental causes. For example, during depression, the frontal cortex will show decreased activation; during mania, temporal lobe regions will show increased activation. Researchers believe that changes in activation can be correlated with blood flow and brain activity. However, we continue to have a limited and rudimentary understanding of the exact mechanisms underlying the disorder. The field is advancing rapidly as findings in brain research and neuroscience expand.

The Role of Genetics

Based on recent research, bipolar disorder is now recognized as an inherited illness where a number of genes interact to make an individual more vulnerable to develop the disorder.[1]

Several respected European adoption studies have found the possibility of developing bipolar disorder to be higher for children who had a birth parent diagnosed with bipolar disorder, whether or not the child was raised with that individual.[2, 3]

When seeing patients, it is very important to ask what other family members may have bipolar disorder, depression, or a history of substance abuse.

Although currently unproven by research, some theorists also suggest that patients may carry the genetic predisposition to bipolar disorder, but not develop symptoms unless exposed to significant stress, especially during developmental periods. For example, extensive substance use or early physical/sexual trauma could trigger this stress-vulnerability.

The Role of Brain Anatomy and Physiology

Brain areas involved with depression and mania include the frontal lobe (where the brain performs many of its executive and organizational functions) and the temporal lobe (involved in regulating emotions). For years, theorists implicated the temporal lobe, which includes the hippocampus and the amygdala, in the development of affective instability, including depression, bipolar disorder, and aggression. For example, those with epilepsy syndromes localized to the temporal lobe (specifically, the hippocampus) develop many bipolar-like symptoms, including unstable moods and paranormal phenomena. Figure 2.1, on the next page, illustrates the specific brain areas impacted by bipolar disorder.

With current neuroimaging technology — PET and SPECT imaging — we can now:

- Identify some brain areas involved in the disorder
- Establish that the brain is physiologically different, depending on the mood state the person is experiencing
- Assess differences in patients' brains when they experience depression versus mania versus euthymia
- Demonstrate how brain function normalizes after medication treatment, indicating that medications effectively return brain activity to more balanced function

Much of the biochemical theory about bipolar disorder stems from our understanding of drug mechanisms, expanding as novel medications have been found effective in the treatment of this illness.

Researchers have learned that interactions producing both abnormal brain states and relative stability are much more complex than originally thought. For example, in evaluating how atypical antipsychotics impact the brain's major neurochemical receptor group, debate continues

Figure 2.1 Brain Areas Impacted by Bipolar Disorder

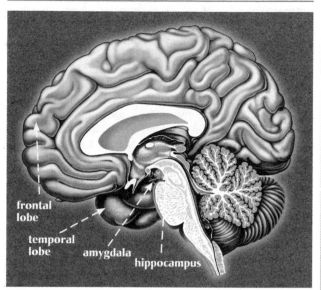

as to whether more serotonin versus less serotonin, more dopamine versus less dopamine (or the combination of the two) are the critical components of mood stabilization.

Research has recently focused on the next level of brain function — secondary messenger systems — neurochemical systems used to carry and communicate activity from a cell's surface throughout the cell body and into areas that determine the cell's genetic products. Our increasing knowledge and understanding of brain function leads to better and more-specific drug development. Observing responses to specific medications likewise informs us regarding brain function and processes.

The Mood Spectrum

Researchers increasingly define the criteria for bipolar disorder as a spectrum of phenotypic manifestations rather than discrete diagnostic phenotypes. Historically, this transition began with Kraepelin's analysis of manic depressive illness as a distinct clinical entity, included within the "greater part of morbid states termed melancholia."[4] Importantly, however, he differentiated patients with "circular" (manic-depressive) forms of melancholia from those without. Lack of clear boundaries between the various mood disorders led many of Kraepelin's successors to continue to "lump patients with manic depressive illness with those who lacked a manic or hypomanic component."[5]

It was not until the 20th century that Leonhard, and subsequently Angst and Perris, reclassified mood disorders into distinct unipolar and bipolar nosological entities. This "split" of mood disorders persists to date and represents a major advance in the approach to patients with mood disorders.

Subsequently, some investigators broadened bipolarity to a dimensional illness, including a spectrum of non-DSM entities [e.g., borderline bipolar, soft bipolar, and affective temperaments (hyperthymic, cyclothymic, dysthymic, irritable)].[5, 6] Akiskal and Pinto emphasized the dimensional nature of the illness by proposing to expand the category to include additional entities and in-between disorders such as bipolar III.[7] The interface of symptoms and "temperament" and implications for course of illness and treatment are active areas of investigation.

The concept of a mood spectrum generally continues to be a topic of debate.

Schizoaffective Disorder: The Continuum Theory

Because patients with bipolar disorder can have psychotic symptoms, one evolving theoretical area views affective disorders (e.g., major depression, bipolar disorder, and

INTRODUCTION

schizophrenia) as a spectrum of disease manifestations, rather than separate disorders with discrete boundaries.[8] Thus, a patient who is predominantly bipolar can have depressive, manic, or psychotic symptoms of variable severity at different time points throughout the course of their disease. Figure 2.2 Continuum of Affective/Psychotic Disorders, below, illustrates this concept.

Patients who manifest both affective and psychotic features are classified as schizoaffective. Schizoaffective disorders, as defined by the DSM-IV(TR), consist of a major depressive, manic, or mixed episode accompanied by delusions or hallucinations that meet the criteria for the diagnosis of schizophrenia.[9] However, the psychotic manifestations must last for at least two weeks after full resolution of the mood symptoms, and the disturbance must not be due to substances of abuse, medications, or a general medical disorder.

PRESENTATION

Figure 2.2 Continuum of Affective/Psychotic Disorders

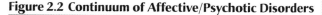

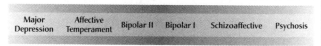

| Major Depression | Affective Temperament | Bipolar II | Bipolar I | Schizoaffective | Psychosis |

CLINICAL PROCESS

The symptoms of schizoaffective disorder share significant features with both bipolar disorder and schizophrenia. Therefore, some investigators have proposed that bipolar disorder and schizophrenia are related members of the schizoaffective continuum and that the predominant manifestation is a function of various genetic and environmental factors. A number of findings support the relationship of the two. For example, both disorders:[10]

PHARMACOTHERAPY

- Have a high degree of genetic transmissibility
- Have certain susceptibility markers that can be co-localized to the same chromosome

RESOURCES

- Reflect similar abnormalities of neurotransmitter systems
- Respond to treatment with newer generation psychotropic (antipsychotic) medications

However, the relationship between the various disorders is still a subject of great debate. Some advocate the unipolar/bipolar dichotomy. Additionally, the genetic basis of these psychiatric diagnoses has not been fully elucidated.

It remains to be seen whether or not a greater understanding of biologic underpinnings will more clearly define a set of discrete disorders or a continuum of disorders.

References for Chapter 2

1. Faraone SV, Glatt SJ, Tsuang MT. The genetics of pediatric-onset bipolar disorder. *Biol Psychiatry.* 2003;53:970–7.

2. Faraone SV, Tsuang MT. Heterogeneity and the genetics of bipolar disorder. *Am J Med Genet.* 2003;123C:1–9.

3. Smoller JW, Finn CT. Family, twin, and adoption studies of bipolar disorder. *Am J Med Genet.* 2003;123C:48–58.

4. Kraepelin E. *Manic Depressive Insanity and Paranoia.* Translated by Barclay RM; edited by Robertson GM. New York: Arno Press: 1976 (originally published 1921).

5. Cassano GB, Frank E, Miniati M, et al. Conceptual underpinnings and empirical support for the mood spectrum. *Psychiatr Clin North Am.* 2002; 25(4):699–712.

6. Angst J. The emerging epidemiology of hypomania and bipolar II disorder. *J Affect Disord.* 1998;50(2-3):143–51.

7. Akiskal HS, Pinto O. The evolving bipolar spectrum. Prototypes I, II, III, and IV. *Psychiatr Clin North Am.* 1999;22(3):517–34, vii.Review.

8. Lapierre YD. Schizophrenia and manic-depression: separate illnesses or a continuum? *Can J Psychiatry.* 1994;39(9 Suppl 2):S59–64.

9. American Psychiatric Association, American Psychiatric Association Task Force on DSM-IV. *Diagnostic and Statistical Manual of Mental Disorders: DSM-IV-TR.* Washington, DC: American Psychiatric Association: 2000.

10. Moller HJ. Bipolar disorder and schizophrenia: distinct illnesses or a continuum? *J Clin Psychiatry.* 2003;64(Suppl 6):23–7; discussion 28.

Chapter 3:
Epidemiology and Risk Factors

Very recent data describes the lifetime and 12-month prevalence rates of bipolar I or II disorder as being 3.9 percent and 2.6 percent, respectively.[1, 2] These studies and others found that bipolar disorder is highly comorbid with numerous anxiety and substance disorders.[2] Overall, research in the last few years indicates an increasing appreciation for the prevalence and severity of bipolar disorder as well as for the symptom persistence and decreased functioning experienced by many.[3, 4]

A number of researchers have identified bipolar disorder as present in about 30 percent of depressed patients in primary care practice.[5–10]

In one very large study that looked at over 85,000 people in the general population, 3.7 percent of the sample screened positive for bipolar disorder with the Mood Disorder Questionnaire (MDQ).[8] When asked about previous diagnoses with mood disorders, responses indicated that, of those who screened positive for bipolar disorder:

> *The MDQ is fundamentally an educational tool for clinicians to use to better discriminate unipolar from bipolar symptoms. Screening positive does not necessarily mean a person has bipolar disorder.[12]*

- Forty-nine percent never received a diagnosis of any mood disorder.
- Twenty percent had previously been diagnosed with bipolar disorder.
- Thirty-one percent had been diagnosed with depression, but not bipolar disorder.

> *Diagnostic delay, misdiagnosis, and unfocused treatment significantly impact those with bipolar disorders.[11]*

Epidemiology

Epidemiologic studies indicate that bipolar disorder is a common and severe psychiatric illness. However, lifelong prevalence is possibly higher than published figures due to:

- Delay between onset of symptoms and diagnosis
- Stigma associated with mental illness
- Some cultural tendency to seek assistance from religious and other, non-medical support systems
- Under-reporting and under-recognition

Much of the problem with under-reporting and under-recognition of bipolar disorder as well as patients being treated with antidepressant monotherapy may stem from:

- The massive effort of the National Institute of Mental Health (NIMH), beginning in 1988, to encourage primary care clinicians to diagnose and treat depression with antidepressants (especially fluoxetine, a "safer" — at least in overdose — antidepressant introduced in 1988). This campaign actually came years before the nature of depression in primary care was adequately characterized.
- The prevalence of bipolar disorder in the primary care clinical population.
- Bipolar disorder's primary expression as depression. Monotherapy antidepressant medication treatment can be harmful: at best, it is not helpful and at worst, for a significant minority, it makes their disorder more acute or chronically worse.[13]

Other factors potentially leading to the overuse of antidepressants in primary care settings include:

- Massive educational efforts that have led to the broad adoption of antidepressants by primary care clinicians with only modest formal exposure to mood disorders in training[14]
- The use of antidepressants among clinicians frequently unfamiliar with mood disorder subtypes

and the need for differential diagnosis prior to treatment attempts

- Antidepressant approvals for various anxiety disorders without an appreciation of the high comorbidity of bipolar disorders with anxiety disorders and anxious or other activated states[15]

Prevalence

It can be difficult to determine the prevalence of bipolar disorder. This is because the diagnosis is not usually established at the time of initial presentation.[16] While mania is clearly a core feature of bipolar I disorder, hypomania (a core feature of bipolar II disorder) may be missed or dismissed as a personality characteristic.

Most patients with bipolar disorder seek help from primary care physicians when they are depressed; thus, a possible diagnosis of bipolar disorder may be overlooked.[17] Consequently, statistics on the incidence of bipolar disorder are retrospective. Frequency statistics generally rely on lifetime prevalence data.

In a population-based, cross-national epidemiologic survey of 38,000 patients from 10 countries, Weissman et al. estimated that the lifetime prevalence of bipolar disorder (as compared to major depression) across countries was:[18]

- More consistent than major depression rates
- Undiagnosed on average for six years before patients seek help, typically for major depression, which can further extend the time from onset to bipolar diagnosis
- Consistent, reflecting the absence of cultural risk factors influencing the epidemiology of major depression

Two major community surveys of the U.S. general population confirmed the findings of Weissman et al.[19, 20] Additional data from the National Comorbidity Study estimated 12-month prevalence at 3.9 percent (with lifetime prevalence at 2.6 percent).[1, 2]

INTRODUCTION

PRESENTATION

CLINICAL PROCESS

PHARMACOTHERAPY

RESOURCES

The American Psychiatric Association suggests that these overall rates of bipolar disorder may be conservative.[21] Hirschfeld et al. utilized the MDQ — a sensitive but non-specific, validated screening tool for bipolar disorder — to determine the potential prevalence of bipolar I, II, and bipolar NOS disorders in the U.S. general population, finding 3.7 percent of the general population screened positive for a possible bipolar disorder.[22] Subsequent research results using such screening measures have been mixed; therefore, these findings are not necessarily indicative of diagnostic prevalence. [12, 23–25]

Gender

The overall incidence of bipolar disorder is approximately gender neutral. However, epidemiological studies indicate that bipolar II disorder, a condition in which depressive episodes predominate, may be somewhat more common in women.[26]

Age of Onset

Although bipolar disorder can present at almost any age, some research indicates a peak period of onset in late adolescence (ages 15–19).[16, 27] Recent research suggests that the age of onset for nearly 33 percent of those with bipolar disorder is under age 13.[28] Thus, it may very well be that a substantial number of individuals with bipolar disorder have experienced diagnostic and treatment delays that adversely impact long-term outcomes.[28]

Onset at the age of 30 years or older appears to be less common; only 16 percent of subjects reported onset of symptoms during this time of their life.[16, 27]

Ethnicity

Although bipolar disorder appears to be no more prevalent among any one ethnic group than another, African Americans with schizoaffective disorders (including the bipolar subtype) are under-diagnosed in favor of schizophrenia or other non-affective psychoses.[29] Some researchers relate this disparity to an interpretative or diagnostic bias identified in the United States, the United Kingdom, and the Caribbean.[30, 31] Others indicate that there may be ethnic differences in clinical presentation that contribute to this disparity.[32]

In recent, large studies of African American and Caucasian patients, African Americans were more likely than other patients to be misdiagnosed as having a schizophrenia spectrum disorder by clinical assessment and structured interview despite no differences in first-rank symptoms from others in the study. The authors surmised that these misdiagnoses might have been due to a perception that the patients' psychotic symptoms were more chronic or persistent than their affective symptoms.[33, 34]

One study found that older African-American patients with bipolar disorder were more likely to be diagnosed with mutually exclusive conditions (e.g., schizophrenia) and risk being under-recognized or misdiagnosed with subsequent inappropriate treatment.[35]

In an eight-month clinical sample of new admissions to a large behavioral health service delivery system, researchers found Latinos to be more likely to receive diagnoses of major depression (rather than bipolar disorder or a schizophrenia spectrum disorder) than other ethnic groups.[36] Possible explanations cited were:

- Self-selection
- Culturally determined expression of symptoms
- Difficulties in accurately applying DSM-IV criteria to Latinos
- Bias related to clinicians' lack of cultural competence
- Inherent lack of precision when using unstructured interviews (possibly combined with clinician bias)

Risk Factors for Bipolar Disorder

A number of variables can influence an individual's risk of clinical manifestations and susceptibility to bipolar disorder, including genetics, physiological/psychological contributors, and environmental contributors.

Genetics

Data from large numbers of family studies as well as adoption studies demonstrate a consistent relationship between family history and risk of bipolar disorder.[37, 38] In family studies, at least two-thirds of patients with bipolar disorder have a family history of affective illness.[38] The risk increases with the presence of major affective illness in parents. If one parent has a major affective disorder, the children have about a 20 percent risk of also being affected.[39] If both parents have an affective disorder, and one is bipolar, the children have a 50 to 75 percent risk of affective illness.[40]

Some of the strongest evidence for the genetic component of bipolar disorder comes from twin studies. Bertelsen et. al. studied a population of 11,288, same-sexed twin pairs born 1870–1920 in Denmark.[41] The study identified 126 probands from 110 pairs and reported concordance rates for bipolar disorder of 62 percent for monozygotic twins and 8 percent for dizygotic twins, resulting in an estimated 59 percent heritability of the disorder for twins.

The exact mode of bipolar disorder inheritance is unknown. Evidence points to susceptibility loci on multiple interacting genes.[42] The strongest evidence supports a role for genes on chromosomes 18p, 18q, and 21q.[43] However, methodological issues make it difficult to convincingly confirm the significance of these loci at this time, due to the fact that they are susceptibility genes, each of which has relatively little influence alone. The genes may either confer susceptibility in limited numbers of families, or sample sizes of various studies are too small to rule out associations by chance alone. Efforts are ongoing to identify and characterize specific susceptibility loci. Recent research indicates that there is an overlap in genetic susceptibility across the mood spectrum and that there are interactions between possible genetic susceptibility and environmental forces.[44, 45]

Among family members with bipolar disorder, the risk for other psychiatric illnesses is significantly elevated as well. For any given individual with bipolar disorder, the likelihood of family members having depression is significant, at least as much as bipolar disorder itself. The risk for other, co-existing psychiatric illnesses is also high, including substance abuse and anxiety disorders. Members of families in which more than one person has bipolar disorder or depression can experience both earlier onset and a more severe course of bipolar disorder.[20, 39]

Physiological and Psychological Contributors

Many medical/physiological diseases/factors can precipitate or exacerbate bipolar disorder manifestations.

Perinatal Complications

There appears to be an association between perinatal complications and risk of psychiatric illness. Several studies describe an association between schizophrenia and obstetrical complications (e.g., degree of parity, maternal bleeding, season of birth).[46, 47] However, the possible association is not as well studied in bipolar disorder.[17, 48]

Reproductive Cycle/Post-Partum Impacts

In women, bipolar disorder can be associated with events of the reproductive cycle and the post-partum state. Of women with bipolar disorder, it is reported that many may experience premenstrual or menstrual exacerbations of mood symptoms, and approximately 25 percent may experience premenstrual depression.[49] Ongoing, prospective studies are expected to provide more hard estimates of the clinical impact of monthly hormonal changes.

INTRODUCTION

PRESENTATION

CLINICAL PROCESS

PHARMACOTHERAPY

RESOURCES

> *It is possible to misdiagnose bipolar disorder as premenstrual dysphoric disorder (PMDD) if one does not take an accurate history and confirm, among other circumstances, that the identified disruption in mood is **only** present during the luteal phase.*

During the post-partum period, women at risk for bipolar disorder face an increased risk of onset; similarly, those in remission face a greater risk of relapse.[50, 51] A 2003 literature review indicated that postpartum (or puerperal) psychosis — a rare disorder often considered a psychiatric emergency — is associated with bipolar disorder.[52] Onset was cited as occurring most often within 48 to 72 hours after childbirth; however, most people develop symptoms within the first 14 days following childbirth. The author noted that this postpartum psychosis requires aggressive treatment to safeguard maternal and neonatal health and well-being.[52] Clinicians will need to balance these safety issues with those associated with the possible teratogenic impact of some medications (typically valproic acid and carbamazepine; however, risks are unknown for the newer anticonvulsants and atypical antipsychotics).[51]

In fact, postpartum psychosis can arise from exacerbations of bipolar illness in the puerperium.[53]

Thyroid Disease Impact

Some patients with thyroid disease may be at increased risk for bipolar disorder, perhaps because thyroid hormone has significant effects on brain metabolism and neural activation. For example, triiodothyronine (T3) may accelerate and augment antidepressant response to tricyclic antidepressants in patients with refractory unipolar depression.[54] Patients with bipolar disorder have been shown to have an increased incidence of antithyroid antibodies compared to controls.[4, 55, 56] In fact, the presence of significant titers of antithyroid antibodies is higher in bipolar patients than in those with other affective disorders.[57]

Cyclothymia

A risk factor for bipolar disorder, episodes characteristic of cyclothymia (fluctuating mood disturbance involving numerous periods of hypomanic and depressive symptoms) are common in patients with bipolar disorder. To determine the clinical course of cyclothymia, Akiskal and colleagues found that the presence of cyclothymic manifestations should be considered indicative that a patient may eventually manifest classical symptoms of bipolar disorder.[58]

Environmental Contributors

Although genetics plays a strong role in the genesis of bipolar disorder, concordance rates less than 100 percent among monozygotic twins support the role of environmental factors as well as more complicated genetic penetrance patterns. It is reasonable to postulate that genetics plays a stronger role in those with early-onset disease.[17]

Studies of socioeconomic influence have been conflicting, alternately suggesting that bipolar disorder is more common in either those of higher or lower socioeconomic status.[16, 59]

Of note, however, are the research results from the Stanley Foundation Study regarding the relationship between early traumatic life events and onset/course of illness for bipolar disorder. That study found that those who experienced physical or sexual abuse as children/adolescents had an earlier age of onset and a more adverse illness course as well as more comorbid psychiatric disorders and incidence of serious suicide attempts.[4]

INTRODUCTION

PRESENTATION

CLINICAL PROCESS

PHARMACOTHERAPY

RESOURCES

References for Chapter 3

1. Kessler RC, Berglund P, Demler O, et al. Lifetime prevalence and age-of-onset distributions of DSM-IV disorders in the National Comorbidity Survey Replication. *Arch Gen Psychiatry*. 2005;62:593–602.

2. Kessler RC, Chiu WT, Demler O, et al. Prevalence, severity, and comorbidity of 12-month DSM-IV disorders in the National Comorbidity Survey Replication. *Arch Gen Psychiatry*. 2005;62:617–27.

3. Judd LL, Askiskal HS, Schettler, PJ, et al. A prospective investigation of the natural history of the long-term weekly symptomatic status of bipolar II disorder. *Arch Gen Psychiatry*. 2003 Mar;60(3):261–9.

4. Post RM, Leverich GS, Altshuler LL, et al. An overview of recent findings of the Stanley Foundation Bipolar Network (Part I). *Bipolar Disord*. 2003;5: 310–19.

5. Manning JS, Haykal RF, Connor PD, et al. On the nature of depressive and anxious states in a family practice setting: the high prevalence of bipolar II and related disorders in a cohort followed longitudinally. *Compr Psychiatry*. 1997 Mar-Apr;38(2):102–8.

6. Manning JS, Zylstra RG, Connor PD. Teaching family physicians about mood disorders: a procedure suite for behavioral medicine. *Prim Care Companion J Clin Psychiatry*. 1999 Feb;1(1):18–23.

7. Coyne JC, Fechner-Bates S, Schwenk TL. Prevalence, nature, and comorbidity of depressive disorders in primary care. *Gen Hosp Psychiatry*. 1994 Jul;16(4):267–76.

8. Hirschfeld RM, Cass AR, Holt DC, et al. Screening for bipolar disorder in patients treated for depression in a family medicine clinic. *J Am Board Fam Pract*. 2005 Jul-Aug;18(4):233–9.

9. Das AK, Olfson M, Gameroff MJ, et al. Screening for bipolar disorder in a primary care practice. *JAMA*. 2005 Feb 23;293(8):956–63.

10. Hirschfeld RM, Calabrese JR, Weissman MM, et al. Screening for bipolar disorder in the community. *J Clin Psychiatry*. 2003 Jan;64(1):53–9.

11. Ghaemi SN, Boiman EE, Goodwin FK. Diagnosing bipolar disorder and the effect of antidepressants: a naturalistic study. *J Clin Psychiatry*. 2000 Oct;61(10):804–8.

12. Phelps JR, Ghaemi SN. Improving the diagnosis of bipolar disorder: predictive value of screening tests. *J Affect Disord*. 2006 Jun;92(2-3):141–8.

13. Regier DA, Hirschfeld RM, Goodwin FK, et al. The NIMH Depression Awareness, Recognition, and Treatment Program: structure, aims, and scientific basis. *Am J Psychiatry*. 1988 Nov;145(11):1351–7.

14. Manning JS, Haykal RF, Akiskal HS. The role of bipolarity in depression in the family practice setting. *Psychiatr Clin North Am*. 1999 Sep;22(3):689–703.

15. Keller MB. Prevalence and impact of comorbid anxiety and bipolar disorder. *J Clin Psychiatry*. 2006;67(Suppl 1):5–7.

16. Bebbington P, Ramana R. The epidemiology of bipolar affective disorder. *Soc Psychiatry Psychiatry Epidemiol*. 1995;30(6):279–92.

17. Rush AJ. Toward an understanding of bipolar disorder and its origin. *J Clin Psychiatry*. 2003;64 (Suppl 6):4–8; discussion 28.

18. Weissman MM, Bland RC, Canino GJ, et al. Cross-national epidemiology of major depression and bipolar disorder. *JAMA*. 1996;276(4):293–9.

19. Regier DA, Farmer ME, Rae DS, et al. Comorbidity of mental disorders with alcohol and other drug abuse. Results from the Epidemiologic Catchment Area (ECA) Study. *JAMA*. 1990;264(19):2511–8.

20. Regier DA, Myers JK, Kramer M, et al. The NIMH Epidemiologic Catchment Area program. Historical context, major objectives, and study population characteristics. *Arch Gen Psychiatry*. 1984;41(10):934–41.

21. American Psychiatric Association: Practice guideline for the treatment of patients with bipolar disorder (revision). *Am J Psychiatry*. 2002;159(Suppl 4):1–50.

22. Hirschfeld RM, Calabrese JR, Weissman MM, et al. Screening for bipolar disorder in the community. *J Clin Psychiatry*. 2003;64(1):53–9.

23. Hirschfeld RM, Holzer C, Calabrese JR, et al. Validity of the Mood Disorder Questionnaire: a general population study. *Am J Psychiatry*. 2003;160:178–80.

24. Hirschfeld RM, Cass AR, Holt DC, et al. Screening for bipolar disorder in patients treated for depression in a family medicine clinic. *J Am Board Fam Pract*. 2005;18:233–9.

25. Miller CJ, Klugman J, Berv DA, et al. Sensitivity and specificity of the Mood Disorder Questionnaire for detecting bipolar disorder. *Journal of Affective Disorders*. 2004;81:167–71.

26. Leibenluft E. Women with bipolar illness: clinical and research issues. *Am J Psychiatry*. 1996;153(2):163–73.

27. Lish JD, Dime-Meenan S, Whybrow PC, et al. The National Depressive and Manic-Depressive Association (DMDA) survey of bipolar members. *J Affect Disord*. 1994;31(4):281–94.

28. Post RM, Kowatch RA. The health care crisis of childhood-onset bipolar illness: some recommendations for its amelioration. *J Clin Psychiatry*. 2006 Jan;67(1):115–25.

29. Blow FC, Zeber JE, McCarthy JF, et al. Ethnicity and diagnostic patterns in veterans with psychoses. *Soc Psychiatry Psychiatr Epidemiol*. 2004;39:841–51.

30. Delbello MP, Soutullo CA, Strakowski SM. Racial differences in treatment of adolescents with bipolar disorder. *Am J Psychiatry*. 2000;157(5):837–8.

INTRODUCTION

PRESENTATION

CLINICAL PROCESS

PHARMACOTHERAPY

RESOURCES

31. Kirov G, Murray RM. Ethnic differences in the presentation of bipolar affective disorder. *Eur Psychiatry.* 1999;14(4):199–204.

32. Kennedy N, Boydell J, van Os J, Murray RM. Ethnic differences in first clinical presentation of bipolar disorder: results from an epidemiological study. *Journal of Affective Disorders.* 2004;83:161–8.

33. Strakowski SM, Keck PE Jr, Arnold LM, et al. Ethnicity and diagnosis in patients with affective disorders. *J Clin Psychiatry.* 2003 Jul;643(7):747–54.

34. Neighbors HW, Trierweiler SJ, Ford BC, et al. Racial differences in DSM diagnosis using a semi-structured instrument: the importance of clinical judgment in the diagnosis of African Americans. *Journal of Health and Social Behavior, Special Issue: Race, Ethnicity, and Mental Health.* 2003 Sept;44(3):237–56.

35. Kilbourne AM, Haas GL, Mulsant BH, et al. Concurrent psychiatric diagnoses by age and race among persons with bipolar disorder. *Psychiatric Services.* 2004;55:931–3.

36. Minsky S, Vega W, Miskimen T, et al. Diagnostic patterns in Latino, African American, and European American psychiatric patients. *Arch Gen Psychiatry.* 2003 Jun;60(6):637–44.

37. Weissman MM, Gershon ES, Kidd KK, et al. Psychiatric disorders in the relatives of probands with affective disorders. The Yale University--National Institute of Mental Health Collaborative Study. *Arch Gen Psychiatry.* 1984;41(1):13–21.

38. Gershon ES, Hamovit J, Guroff JJ, et al. A family study of schizoaffective, bipolar I, bipolar II, unipolar, and normal control probands. *Arch Gen Psychiatry.* 1982;39(10):1157–67.

39. Todd RD, Geller B, Neuman R, et al. Increased prevalence of alcoholism in relatives of depressed and bipolar children. *J Am Acad Child Adolesc Psychiatry.* 1996;35(6):716–24.

40. Potter W. Biological findings in bipolar disorders, in *Annual Review. vol 6.* Edited by Hales R, American Psychiatric Association; 1987.

41. Bertelsen A, Harvald B, Hauge M. A Danish twin study of manic-depressive disorders. *Br J Psychiatry.* 1977;130:330–51.

42. Craddock N, Khodel V, Van Eerdewegh P, et al. Mathematical limits of multilocus models: the genetic transmission of bipolar disorder. *Am J Hum Genet.* 1995; 57(3):690–702.

43. NIMH Genetics Workgroup. *Genetics and mental disorders.* NIH Publication No. 98-4268. Rockville, MD: National Institute of Mental Health, 1998.

44. Craddock N, Forty L. Genetics of affective (mood) disorders. *European Journal of Human Genetics.* 2006;14:660–8.

45. Payne JL, Potash JB, DePaulo JR Jr. Recent findings on the genetic basis of bipolar disorder. *Psychiatr Clin N Am.* 2005;28:481–98.

46. Schwarzkopf SB, Nasrallah HA, Olson SC, et al. Perinatal complications and genetic loading in schizophrenia: preliminary findings. *Psychiatry Res.* 1989;27(3):233–9.

47. Hultman CM, Sparen P, Takei N, et al. Prenatal and perinatal risk factors for schizophrenia, affective psychosis, and reactive psychosis of early onset: case-control study. *BMJ.* 1999;318(7181):421–6.

48. Kinney DK, Yurgelun-Todd DA, Tohen M. Pre- and perinatal complications and risk for bipolar disorder: a retrospective study. *J Affect Disord.* 1998;50(2-3):117–24.

49. Arnold LM. Gender differences in bipolar disorder. *Psychiatr Clin North Am.* 2003;26(3):595–620.

50. Hunt N, Silverstone T. Does puerperal illness distinguish a subgroup of bipolar patients? *J Affect Disord.* 1995;34(2):101–7.

51. Viguera AC, Cohen LS, Baldessarini RJ, et al. Managing bipolar disorder during pregnancy: weighing the risks and benefits. *Can J Psychiatry.* 2002 June;47(5):426–36.

52. Cohen LS. Gender-specific considerations in the treatment of mood disorders in women across the life cycle. *J Clin Psychiatry.* 2003;64(suppl 15):18–29.

53. Chaudron LH, Pies RW. The relationship between postpartum psychosis and bipolar disorder: a review. *J Clin Psychiatry.* 2003;64:1284–92.

54. Bauer M, Whybrow PC. Thyroid hormone, neural tissue and mood modulation. *World J Biol Psychiatry.* 2001;2(2):59–69.

55. Haggerty JJ Jr, Evans DL, Golden RN, et al. The presence of antithyroid antibodies in patients with affective and nonaffective psychiatric disorders. *Biol Psychiatry.* 1990;27(1):51–60.

56. Haggerty JJ Jr, Silva SG, Marquardt M, et al. Prevalence of antithyroid antibodies in mood disorders. *Depression and Anxiety.* 1997;5:91–6.

57. Oomen HA, Schipperijn AJ, Drexhage HA. The prevalence of affective disorder and in particular of a rapid cycling of bipolar disorder in patients with abnormal thyroid function tests. *Clin Endocrinol (Oxf).* 1996;45(2):215–23.

58. Akiskal HS, Djenderedjian AM, Rosenthal RH, et al. Cyclothymic disorder: validating criteria for inclusion in the bipolar affective group. *Am J Psychiatry.* 1977;134(11):1227–33.

59. Verdoux H, Bourgeois M. Social class in unipolar and bipolar probands and relatives. *J Affect Disord.* 1995;33(3):181–7.

INTRODUCTION

PRESENTATION

CLINICAL PROCESS

PHARMACOTHERAPY

RESOURCES

Chapter 4:
The Patient with Depression

Helping patients with symptoms of depression can present a significant diagnostic conundrum for clinicians — how to differentiate major depression from the depressed phase of bipolar disorder. Patients struggling with sadness, sleep problems, diminished interest in activities they used to enjoy, inability to function effectively at work, relationship problems — all the hallmarks of depression — will often seek help from their primary care physician or other health care professional. Patients experiencing manic or hypomanic symptoms are far less likely to seek professional help during those episodes.

Further complicating this conundrum are the impacts of misdiagnosis: antidepressant monotherapy, at best, will be ineffective for a person with bipolar depression. At worst, it may likely propel the patient into more significant manic/hypomanic suffering (or mixed presentation) with increased suffering and potentially lethal, long-term outcomes.

> *Clearly, differentiating unipolar from bipolar depression is vital, requiring that unipolar major depression become a diagnosis of exclusion.*

Bipolar depression significantly impacts a person's ability to function and is perhaps the most difficult expression of bipolar illness to treat. Research indicates that these episodes tend to be more frequent and long-lasting than manic ones.[1-3] Of significant concern is the greater risk of attempted and completed suicide among those suffering from bipolar depression over mania.[4-6] Long-term data suggests that patients may experience some degree of subsyndromal depressive symptoms greater than 30 percent of the time.[3]

SECTION B: THE PATIENT WITH BIPOLAR DISORDER – INITIAL PRESENTATION

To establish a foundation for identifying and treating patients with bipolar depression, this chapter provides information on:

- Initial presentation of patients who are depressed and may be suffering from bipolar disorder
- Recognizing symptoms of depression
- DSM-IV(TR) criteria for major depression
- Suicide risk in bipolar depression
- Characteristics of depressive mixed states often seen with bipolar illness

Initial Presentation

The following represents information about two patients — Holly and Bill — who visit their primary care physician with symptoms that could be related to either unipolar or bipolar depression.

HOLLY

Holly is 35 years old and suffers from migraines, which is what prompted her to make the appointment today. These headaches are a common problem for her, causing frequent visits to emergency rooms and urgent care facilities. Sitting slumped over on the exam table, Holly appears very sad, talking and moving slowly. When asked about her sadness, she replied that her ". . . headaches were depressing all by themselves!" She does admit to having been treated often in the past for depression and panic attacks.

For the migraine, she had tried two doses of a "triptan" medication used for rescue, but without relief. She used over-the-counter medications frequently for both headache and insomnia. Her medication list included an inhaled corticosteroid and albuterol-metered dose inhaler (used once or twice monthly) for moderate persistent asthma as well as clonazepam prescribed "prn" for anxiety. She is married (her second) and had a tubal ligation after the birth of her second child.

There's obviously a lot going on with Holly: her migraines don't seem to respond to treatment, she suffers from insomnia that appears difficult to remedy, she's been treated for both depressive symptoms and anxiety in the past, and has some evidence of dysfunction in relationships. Family and psychiatric history will be very important in assessing her level of suffering and possible causes.

BILL

Bill is 51 years old when he visits an urgent care facility with a chief complaint of depressed mood. "This is the worst one I can remember," he comments. In the interview, he describes having experienced a three- to four-year period during which he had not felt his mood was ever normal. Although his daughter had died tragically four years before, he still experienced "unrelenting sadness" for several weeks at a time and extremely low motivation. "Right now, I don't care about anything. I feel 'dead' inside," he said. "I'd rather feel sad than be without any feelings at all." Bill, an articulate man, looks sad and sits in the exam room chair while resting his upper body on the counter beside him, head in hand – a typical melancholic posture.

Bill appears to be experiencing major depression that has lasted much longer than typical bereavement over his daughter's death. It will be critical to find out about Bill's family history, what happened to his daughter, and any psychiatric history prior to her death that may provide more insight into what's associated with his current suffering **before** selecting treatment modalities.

The next section, Bipolar Illness Clinical Process — A Patient-Focused Approach, *follows both Holly and Bill through the clinical process of assessment and differential diagnosis, establishing a working diagnosis and therapeutic relationships, selecting treatment modalities, and managing the illness.*

INTRODUCTION

PRESENTATION

CLINICAL PROCESS

PHARMACOTHERAPY

RESOURCES

Recognizing Symptoms of Depression

A major depressive episode is characterized by depressed mood or loss of interest or pleasure in previously enjoyed activities for a period of at least two weeks.

Additionally, the individual may experience some or all of the following:

- Increased or decreased need for sleep
- Increased or decreased appetite
- Loss of energy
- Difficulty initiating action/behavior
- Diminished ability to concentrate
- Social withdrawal
- Feelings of worthlessness
- Thoughts of suicide or death

In children and adolescents, the predominant mood may be irritable rather than sad, accompanied by additional symptoms from the list above.

When they are depressed, people with bipolar disorder are often profoundly sad, irritable, or in a "numb" mood. They may report that life is totally without pleasure and not worth living, despite acknowledging positive things that "should" help them feel happy or satisfied. During depression, people lose interest and enjoyment in their usual activities, including basic pleasures, such as eating and having sex.

The experience of clinically significant depression goes far beyond an everyday sad feeling.

Core depression symptoms involve changes in sleeping and eating habits. Many find it difficult to fall asleep, waking up several times each night and earlier in the morning than desired. About 20 percent of people sleep more when depressed than they normally do when not experiencing depression. In all cases, those experiencing depression awaken without feeling rested. Changes in appetite can be determined by a corresponding weight loss or an increase in appetite, without necessarily feeling the food they eat is satisfying or appealing.

Those with depression often have difficulty with concentration, memory, and decision-making. There is impairment in the person's social and/or occupational functioning.

Minor depressive symptoms and anxiety can precede a major depressive episode by weeks or months. Onset of major depressive symptoms generally occurs over a period of days or weeks; an untreated episode usually lasts four or more months.

Diagnostic Criteria for Major Depression

Major depression is the most acutely severe, depressive mood disorder. Figure 4.1, below and on the following page, lists the diagnostic criteria for major depression, which may be the patient's sole mood disorder (unipolar depression) **or** a component of a bipolar disorder.

This information on major depressive disorder provides a foundation for identifying and treating patients with bipolar disorder who may initially present with depressive symptoms. It is important that a diagnosis of major depressive disorder be one of exclusion, ruling out the possibility of bipolar disorder first.

Figure 4.1   Criteria for Major Depressive Episodes[7]

A. Five (or more) of the following symptoms have been present during the same 2-week period and represent a change from previous functioning; at least one of the symptoms is either (1) depressed mood or (2) loss of interest or pleasure. **Note:** Do not include symptoms that are clearly due to a general medical condition, or mood-incongruent delusions or hallucinations.

  1. Depressed mood most of the day, nearly every day, as indicated by either subjective report (e.g., feels sad or empty) or observation made by others (e.g., appears tearful). **Note:** in children and adolescents, can be irritable mood.

  2. Markedly diminished interest or pleasure in all, or almost all, activities most of the day, nearly every day (as indicated by either subjective account or observation made by others).

  3. Significant weight loss without a diet, weight gain over five percent of body weight in a month, or decreased/increased

(continued)

Figure 4.1   (continued)

appetite nearly every day. **Note:** in children, consider failure to achieve expected weight gains.

4. Insomnia or hypersomnia nearly every day.

5. Psychomotor agitation or retardation nearly every day (observable by others, not merely subjective feelings of restlessness or being slowed down).

6. Fatigue or loss of energy nearly every day.

7. Feelings of worthlessness or excessive/inappropriate guilt (may be delusional) nearly every day (not merely self-reproach or guilt about being sick).

8. Diminished ability to think, concentrate, or be decisive, nearly every day (either by subjective account or as observed by others).

9. Recurrent thoughts of death (not just fear of dying), recurrent suicidal ideation without a specific plan, or a suicide attempt or a specific plan for committing suicide.

B. The symptoms do not meet criteria for a Mixed Episode (see text).

C. The symptoms cause clinically significant distress or impairment in social, occupational, or other important areas of functioning.

D. The symptoms are not due to the direct physiological effects of a substance (e.g., a drug of abuse, a medication) or a general medical condition (e.g., hypothyroidism).

E. The symptoms are not better accounted for by bereavement (i.e., after the loss of a loved one, the symptoms persist for longer than two months or are characterized by marked functional impairment, morbid preoccupation with worthlessness, suicidal ideation, psychotic symptoms, or psychomotor retardation).

Reprinted with permission of American Psychiatric Association, Diagnostic and Statistical Manual of Mental Disorders, Fourth Edition, Text Revision, Washington, D.C., American Psychiatric Association, 2000.

INTRODUCTION

PRESENTATION

CLINICAL PROCESS

PHARMACOTHERAPY

RESOURCES

Dysthymia and depression NOS are two other types of depressive disorders defined in the DSM-IV(TR).[7] Dysthymia is a low-intensity, chronic mood disorder of two or more years' duration. Characteristic features include anhedonia, low self esteem, and low energy. Depression NOS is also referred to as minor depression because the number of symptoms are less than those required for major depression. Interestingly, in primary care practices, 10 to 18 percent of patients with depression NOS will develop a major depressive disorder within a year.[8, 9]

Suicide Risk in Bipolar Depression

Bipolar disorder is accompanied by a high risk for self-injury and suicide when untreated or when patients experience limited response to treatment.[10, 11]

Those with comorbid alcohol or substance abuse or dependence are at greater risk for suicide, as are those who have made previous suicide attempts. There are multiple assessment tools designed to

Assessment of suicide risk is a complex and multidimensional task, and should be an ongoing aspect of interactions between care providers and the patient.

assist clinicians in assessing suicide risk. Most of these include some assessment of these general domains:

- The wish to live or die
- Experience of impulses related to suicide as well as control over these impulses
- Duration and frequency of suicidal ideation (thoughts)
- Specificity of ideas or plans for suicide
- Access to lethal means

Untreated, lengthy periods of severe depression can lead to thoughts about or actual attempts to commit suicide, making treatment particularly critical for those with bipolar disorder.

- Deterrents to suicide (e.g., support from family members, religious beliefs)
- Any active preparation for suicide (e.g., writing letters to loved ones, giving away dear possessions)

Characteristics of Depressive Mixed States

Syndromal depressions that contain significant admixtures of manic symptoms have been termed depressive mixed states (DMX) or mixed/dysphoric hypomania. Such states have been recognized historically with various nomenclatures attached. Kraepelin described several variations including melancholia agitata or activa as well as depression with flight of ideas. The propensity of such states to include intense anxiety led Kraepelin to use the term, "Angstmelancholie," as well.[12]

There is a continuum of symptoms that make up a mixed state, ranging from hypomanic and sub-syndromal depressive symptoms to a full mixed episode as defined by DSM-IV(TR) criteria (see page 62), which involves full DSM-defined symptoms of mania and major depressive disorder being present at the same time.

> *Chapter 5 includes characteristics and DSM-IV (TR) criteria for mixed episodes, focusing on those where mania (rather than hypomania) becomes fully mixed with a major depressive episode (rather than sub-syndromal depressive symptoms).*

Characteristics of depressive mixed states include:

- Racing thoughts that often inhibit initiation of sleep
- Noticeably increased activity usually present well into the early morning hours (e.g., cleaning, rearranging furniture, and intense involvement in various projects both creative and otherwise)
- Tone of increased activity is often one of pessimism and dissatisfaction with brooding
- Irritability and agitation that may easily be excused as nonspecific expressions of major depression

- Grandiose mood, often manifested toward others in demanding tones with an insistence that others serve the agenda of the patient (not present in "unipolar" major depression)
- Sexual excitement (also not present in "unipolar" major depression)

All of these features might be brought about or accentuated by antidepressant monotherapies. In addition, without a clear picture that the clinician is dealing with a bipolar mixed state, such symptoms could prompt the initiation of anxiolytics or sedative/hypnotics, further complicating the patient's suffering and potential for effective, timely bipolar treatment.

Patients experiencing symptoms of mixed states differ significantly from those with pure mania. As a result, one must remain alert with patients presenting with depression; hypomanic or manic symptoms can co-occur but be episodic and unrecognized by the patient as a change in state.

When manic energy drives excitement or restless anxiety into a depression, the clinical picture becomes ripe for a misdiagnosis of agitated depression, panic disorder, or generalized anxiety disorder. It is therefore important to consider the possibility of bipolar disorder in patients who present pleomorphic illness of this type. Figure 4.2, on the next page, describes the features of this common clinical scenario. Practitioner education on the necessity to consider course, temperament, and family history when treating depression may improve bipolar spectrum disorder identification and limit the use of unproductive or potentially harmful antidepressant monotherapy.

INTRODUCTION

PRESENTATION

CLINICAL PROCESS

PHARMACOTHERAPY

RESOURCES

Figure 4.2   Features of a Depressive Mixed State

Clinical Observations	Patient Complaints	Reports of Significant Others
Depressed mood	Anxiety, including panic states; often refractory	Irascibility
Psychic agitation	Inner tension	Continuous complaining
Dramatic gestures and facial expressions	Muscle tension	Occasional sexual hyperactivity
Restlessness	Pronounced irritability with capacity for rage	Restless activity
Talkativeness	Racing or crowded thoughts	
Emotional lability	Initial or middle insomnia	
Impulsivity – including suicide attempts	Suicidal ideas and impulses	

Adapted from Koukopoulos and Koukopoulos 1999.[13]

References for Chapter 4

1. Hirschfeld RM. Bipolar depression: the real challenge. *Eur Neuropsycho Pharmacol*. 2004;14(suppl 2):83–8.

2. Calabrese JR, Hirschfeld RM, Frye MA, et al. Impact of depressive symptoms compared with manic symptoms in bipolar disorder: results of a U.S. community-based sample. *J Clin Psychiatry*. 2004;65:1499–504.

3. Judd LL, Akiskal HS, Schettler PJ, et al. The long-term natural history of the weekly symptomatic status of bipolar I disorder. *Arch Gen Psychiatry*. 2002;59:530–7.

4. Isometsa ET, Henriksson MM, Aro HM, et al. Suicide in bipolar disorder in Finland. *Am J Psychiatry*. 1994;151:1020–4.

5. Kupfer DJ, Frank E, Grochocinski VJ, et al. Demographic and clinical characteristics of individuals in a bipolar disorder case registry. *J Clin Psychiatry*. 2002;63:120–5.

6. Tondo L, Isacsson G, Baldessarini R. Suicial behaviour in bipolar disorder: risk and prevention. *CNS Drugs*. 2003;17:491–511.

7. American Psychiatric Association, American Psychiatric Association Task Force on DSM-IV. *Diagnostic and Statistical Manual of Mental Disorders: DSM-IV-TR*. Washington, DC: American Psychiatric Association; 2000.

8. Maier W, Gansicke M, Weiffenbach O. The relationship between major and subthreshold variants of unipolar depression. *J Affect Disord*. 1997;45(1-2):41–51.

9. Wells KB, Stewart A, Hays RD, et al. The functioning and well-being of depressed patients. Results from the Medical Outcomes Study. *JAMA*. 1989; 262(7):914–9.

10. Dilsaver SC, Chen YW, Swann AC, et al. Suicidality in patients with pure and depressive mania. *Am J Psychiatry*. 1994;151:1312–15.

11. Strakowski SM, McElroy SL, Keck Jr. PE, West SA. Suicidality among patients with mixed and manic bipolar disorder. *Am J Psychiatry*. 1996,153:674–6.

12. Kraepelin E. *Psychiatrae, ed 5*. Leipzig: JA. Barth; 1896.

13. Koukopoulos A, Koukopoulos A. Agitated depression as a mixed state and the problem of melancholia. *Psychiatr Clin North Am*. 1999 Sep;22(3):547–64.

INTRODUCTION

PRESENTATION

CLINICAL PROCESS

PHARMACOTHERAPY

RESOURCES

Chapter 5:
The Patient with Hypomania/ Mania or Mixed Episodes

Hypomania is a mood state manifested by persistently elevated, expansive, or irritable mood that affects, but does not severely compromise, an individual's functioning at home or at work. Mania, on the other hand, is usually far more evident as it is severely dysfunctional and more intense and troublesome to the patient and everyone around them. Essentially, DSM-IV(TR) characterizes hypomanic symptoms as different from manic symptoms in terms of **duration** (persisting at least four days versus one week for mania) and **intensity** (insufficient to produce marked social or occupational impairment or require hospitalization as can be typical with patients suffering from mania).

A common phenomena in bipolar illness involves mixed episodes, where mania is mixed with symptoms of major depressive disorder. Mixed or dysphoric hypomania — a mixture of hypomania and either DSM-defined or subsyndromal major depressive disorder symptoms (as discussed in chapter 4) — is particularly common in women and can result in severe dysfunction and risk of suicide.[1]

This chapter presents information on:

- The initial presentation of patients who may be suffering from hypomanic and/or manic symptoms
- How to recognize symptoms of hypomania and mania
- DSM-IV criteria for mania (note that DSM defines hypomania as having the same criteria as mania except for duration and intensity of symptoms)
- Characteristics of DSM-IV(TR) mixed episodes

Initial Presentation

The following represents information about two patients — Holly (first introduced in chapter 4) and Janice — who visit their primary care physician with symptoms that could be related to either hypomania or mania.

HOLLY

Holly's husband mentions that there are times when he can do nothing right, and she is highly critical of others: he can't cheer her up, and she may complain of sadness, but her restlessness is more apparent. During these times, it's hard to distract her from what's bothering her, help her get things done to her satisfaction, or even figure out what's bothering her. He's amazed that she seems so full of energy to clean and organize around the house but acts so incredibly sad. Holly has gained some weight since her last visit, admitting that her ". . . current drug of choice is food." When she's feeling depressed, she confesses to binging on chocolate and desserts. In the past, she has used alcohol binges to "unwind" or to sleep. She still suffers from panic attacks but uses her clonazepam if she feels one coming on.

Upon further questioning of both Holly and her husband during the initial visit, the physician learns that this marriage is under a great deal of stress and both parties are looking for answers. When asked about the binge eating, Holly recounts only using purging once in high school. Queried about the panic attacks, she reports that the antidepressants she's been given in the past have really done nothing for her panic attacks — even making them worse on occasion.

JANICE

Janice is 28 years old when she visits her primary care physician, declaring: "I need to take a leave of absence!" She held short-term disability and Family Medical Leave Act (FMLA) papers in hand. A close friend accompanied her and was in the waiting room in case she was needed to provide more information.

INTRODUCTION

Janice works as a customer service representative and has had a number of recent confrontations with co-workers and her supervisor. She had been threatened with dismissal and advised to contact the Employee Assistance Program (EAP) immediately. Janice was noticeably restless and over-active. Her speech was rapid. She got up on one occasion to pace the room.

Asked to describe her situation and symptoms, Janice replied, "I'm losing control. Nothing is going right for me. I'm always angry, and there's nothing I can do about it." Janice began to cry, and asked, "Can my friend come in with me?"

Her friend explained that Janice's family and friends were quite concerned about her recent behavior. Over the last month, Janice had become increasingly argumentative. Her drinking, an episodic problem in the past with one conviction for driving under the influence, had escalated.

PRESENTATION

Her moods seemed erratic to others, her friend explained. One day she could be laughing and going on spending sprees at the mall; the next she might be screaming at trivial matters or crying and complaining that she would be better off dead. Janice had been calling others in the middle of the night to complain about how others were planning to get her fired and sabotaging her work. "She'd have been fired already, if she weren't friends with her supervisor and number one in productivity during the last quarter at work," the friend said.

CLINICAL PROCESS

Janice is clearly experiencing a crisis period in her life. She is too upset to tell a coherent story. Without the accompanying friend, it would be difficult to assess impairment, risk to self/others, and observable behaviors that might be important.

PHARMACOTHERAPY

The next section, Bipolar Illness Clinical Process — A Patient-Focused Approach, *follows both Holly and Janice through the clinical process of assessment and differential diagnosis, establishing a working diagnosis and therapeutic relationships, selecting treatment modalities, and managing their illness.*

RESOURCES

Recognizing Symptoms of Hypomania

Hypomania resembles mania, but does not meet full DSM-IV(TR) criteria for a manic episode. When experiencing a "pure" or "euphoric" hypomanic mood, individuals report feeling on top of things, productive, sociable, and self-confident. They feel excited, energized, creative, active, intelligent, and sometimes, more sexual. They may say that they feel better than at any other time in their lives, and fail to recognize errors in judgment, neglect of everyday duties, or other subtle lapses in functioning. They cannot understand why anyone would call their experience abnormal or part of a disorder.

Because of this perception, one of the criteria for diagnosing hypomania is a change of state observable by others. Verifying this noticeable change of state can best be done by talking with family members or close associates who can comment on previous behavior.

The hypomanic mood can also be accompanied by additional symptoms:

- Inflated self-esteem or grandiosity
- Less need for sleep (manifested by waking earlier)

> *Hypomanic manifestations must not be secondary to the effects of medications, substances of abuse, or a general medical condition. Psychotic symptoms occurring during hypomania automatically define the episode as mania.*[2]

- Pressured speech or being talkative and/or distinctly more social
- Flight of ideas
- Distractibility characterized by rapid changes in speech or activities in response to irrelevant external stimuli
- Increased mental/physical activity, especially of a creative/productive, goal-directed nature; or psychomotor agitation
- Excessive involvement in pleasurable and high-risk activities (that are less impulsive/destructive in nature than in mania)
- Having a tendency for impaired social judgment

These "pure" or "euphoric" episodes appear to be less common than a "mix" of hypomanic and depressive symptoms that fail to meet the threshold for a defined depressive episode (see chapter 4, pages 41 through 42). In women, this "dysphoric" hypomania may be experienced as increased irritability, anger, or sadness in conjunction with extra physical and mental energy.[1] Men may present differently, with more irritable/agitated depression that can stem from bipolar illness.[1] See pages 61 through 63 for a more detailed discussion of mixed episodes where hypomanic symptoms occur along with those of DSM-defined major depressive disorder.

The occurrence, duration, and recurrence of hypomanic episodes are different than those of mania or depression. Hypomanic episodes tend to be briefer and more transient than mania; they may begin and end abruptly. Hypomania can also be inter-episodic and intra-episodic (arising during a depressive episode) with the characteristics of the hypomanic mood strongly influenced by the pre-existence of depression as an energized depressed mood often appears predominately irritable.

When elated mood predominates at onset, it can deteriorate into irritable mood later in

Between five and 15 percent of patients with hypomania later develop a manic or mixed episode.[2]

the episode. This propensity for mood and psychomotor energy to be out of phase (move in opposite directions) is a prevalent, yet often under-appreciated, characteristic to be aware of when evaluating bipolar disorder.

The illustration in figure 5.1, on page 54, indicates that:

1. Hypomania often appears as an abrupt switch out of syndromal or sub-syndromal depressive symptomatology.

2. Such switches often appear on arising or late in the evening.

3. Mood may be elated or irritable.

4. Usual duration is one to three days despite DSM criteria threshold of minimum four days.[3-6]

INTRODUCTION

PRESENTATION

CLINICAL PROCESS

PHARMACOTHERAPY

RESOURCES

Figure 5.1   Bipolar II Hypomanic Episode

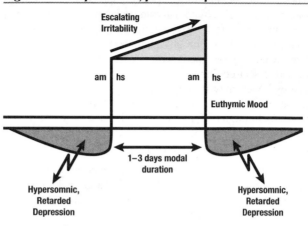

Although DSM-IV(TR) defines a hypomanic episode as a distinct period of persistently elevated, expansive, or irritable mood lasting at least four days, research indicates that symptoms occurring from one to three days can be indicative of hypomania as well.[3–6] For example, there is abundant evidence that a two-day criterion would improve sensitivity without sacrificing specificity.[4,7] Also, a temperament trait of mood lability may better predict bipolar outcome than DSM-IV(TR) hypomanic episodes in depressed patients when followed longitudinally.[8]

Hypomania may be under-reported by patients for a variety of reasons. The patient may not remember or recognize hypomanic symptoms because they:

- Lack needed psychoeducation about the illness and symptoms that are "red flags" for mood episodes
- Suffer from impaired memory due to a depressive episode
- Perceive the experience during a hypomanic episode as essentially positive

The detection of hypomania enables physicians to diagnose the most subtle forms of bipolar disorder. A careful search for such periods of abnormal mood is, therefore, a critical step in the process of differential diagnosis. (See chapter 7 for detailed information on differential diagnosis.)

Recognizing Symptoms of Mania

A manic episode is defined by a distinct period of persistently elevated, expansive, or irritable mood lasting at least one week (or less if hospitalization is required). When manic, some patients experience symptoms of psychosis (including delusions and hallucinations), indicating being out of touch with reality in certain important ways.

Manic symptoms can appear as:

- **A highly excited, energetic mood state** — Feeling "on top of the world" and able to achieve anything despite a decreased ability to complete necessary tasks or tend to daily functions. Those with mania feel they need very little sleep or rest. They may spend excessively, participate in indiscriminate social/sexual interactions, or act impulsively. While the manic individual may feel happy and expansive, friends and family will recognize their behavior as excessive, and may refer the person for treatment. Untreated, mania will worsen, with moods becoming more elevated or irritable, behavior more unpredictable, and judgment more impaired. When manic, patients are often unaware of the consequences of extreme behavior due to confusion, disorientation, and loss of contact with reality.

- **An irritable, excited mood** — Moods fluctuate between euphoria and irritability, all charged by excessive energy, restlessness, and agitation. The patient will have a subjective sense of racing thoughts and, while initiating many projects, will finish few.

Onset of a manic episode is usually sudden and may follow psychosocial stressors. Following onset, symptoms rapidly increase over the next several days. Bipolar disorder's clinical course is recurrent: once a manic episode occurs, more than 90 percent of patients will have additional episodes. Without treatment, episodes tend to occur at 1- to 2.5-year intervals.

Approximately 10 to 15 percent of adolescents with a history of recurrent major depressive episodes eventually present with a manic episode.[2]

Although manic episodes can occur in children and seniors, the mean age range for onset is in the late teens to early 20s.[9]

Diagnostic Criteria for Mania

Although classified as a syndrome of mood disturbance, mania is also characterized by alterations in behavior, cognition, and perception.[10] Figure 5.2 Criteria for Manic Episodes, on page 57, lists the DSM-IV(TR) criteria (criteria A–E) for a manic episode. Following the criteria listing, figure 5.3, on page 58, provides example manifestations of each of the key criterion B symptoms.

Rather than the stereotypical sustained period of euphoria and grandiosity, manic mood symptoms can vary in severity

Failing to recognize that manic manifestations are not all euphoric can potentially result in a missed diagnosis.

from one person to another. Whether or not euphoric in nature, mania must, however, significantly impact functional domains. Examples of such impact include:

- Participating in illegal behavior
- Failing to recognize consequences of foolish business decisions
- Exhibiting unusual sexual behavior
- Threatening others

To meet DSM-IV(TR) criteria, manic symptoms must persist for at least one week. However, if the functional impairment requires hospitalization, the criteria allows for less than one week's duration. The need for hospitalization or presence of psychotic manifestations also meets criterion D for marked impairment.

Figure 5.2   Criteria for Manic Episodes[2]

A.   A distinct period of abnormally and persistently elevated, expansive, or irritable mood, lasting at least one week (or any duration if hospitalization is necessary).

B.   During the period of mood disturbance, three (or more) of the following symptoms have persisted (four if the mood is only irritable) and have been present to a significant degree:

1. Inflated self-esteem or grandiosity

2. Decreased need for sleep (e.g., feels rested after only three hours of sleep)

3. More talkative than usual or pressure to keep talking

4. Flight of ideas or subjective experience that thoughts are racing

5. Distractibility (i.e., attention too easily drawn to unimportant or irrelevant external stimuli)

6. Increase in goal-directed activity (either socially, at work or school, or sexually) or psychomotor agitation

7. Excessive involvement in pleasurable activities that have a high potential for painful consequences (e.g., engaging in unrestrained buying sprees, sexual indiscretions, or foolish business investments)

C.   The symptoms do not meet criteria for a Mixed Episode.

D.   The mood disturbance is sufficiently severe to cause marked impairment in occupational functioning or in usual social activities or relationships with others, or to necessitate hospitalization to prevent harm to self or others, or there are psychotic features.

E.   The symptoms are not due to the direct physiological effects of a substance (e.g., drug of abuse, a medication, or other treatment) or a general medical condition (e.g., hyperthyroidism).

Reprinted with permission of American Psychiatric Association, Diagnostic and Statistical Manual of Mental Disorders, Fourth Edition, Text Revision, Washington, D.C., American Psychiatric Association, 2000.

Figure 5.3   Criterion B Manic Features

B Criterion	Example Manifestations
B1 — Inflated Self Esteem	• Trying to advise public figures, inventing things that defy physics • Being irritable/angry with those not convinced of one's perceptions of self-worth/grandeur
B2 — Less Sleep Needs	• Waking with excess energy, earlier than usual • Going days without sleep but not fatigued
B3 — Pressured Speech	• Speaking in a rapid, loud, difficult-to-understand, ongoing, and hard-to-interrupt manner • Being prone to monologues outside awareness • Making grandiose gestures/wordplay; singing • Haranguing others, complaining, making hostile statements (when mood is irritable, not expansive)
B4 — Flight of Ideas	• Rapidly expressing continuous idea stream • Switching topics suddenly • Being incoherent or completely disorganized
B5 — Distractibility	• Focusing suddenly on discussion across the room (when in conversation) • Focusing on extraneous stimuli, such as the speaker's hair or clothes, during conversation • Interrupting others with irrelevant thoughts
B6 — Increase in Goal-Directed Activity	• Writing multiple letters to convey perceptions to friends and public figures • Calling friends or strangers any time, day or night, without concern for intrusion • Starting projects without finishing others
B7 — Impulsive Pursuit of High-Risk Activities	• Excessively spending beyond income means • Engaging in unprotected sex with strangers • Driving recklessly

Associated Features of Mania

When an individual is manic or experiencing a mixed episode, mood alterations may fluctuate widely — the patient may be euphoric one day and dysphoric the next. Alternately, a depressed period may last for minutes or hours and may occur simultaneously with mania.

Although the typical expansive, cheerful, or euphoric mood of those experiencing mania may have an infectious quality for strangers, those who know the patient recognize it as excessive.

As described, mania manifestations include mood alterations as specified in the DSM-IV(TR). Other disturbances in behavior and cognition often associated with mania are indicated in figure 5.4 on the next page.

Disruptive behavior of various kinds warrants consideration of bipolar illness. When manic, patients can also exhibit some antisocial behavior, disregard ethical boundaries, physically threaten others, or attempt suicide. However, suicidal thoughts are more likely to occur during a mixed rather than a classic manic episode.[11] See pages 61 through 63 for a description of mixed manic/hypomanic episodes.

As mania develops, patients may:

- Abuse substances (e.g., alcohol, stimulants), which may worsen or prolong the episode
- Experience significant impairments in their relationships with spouses or partners, other family members, fellow employees, or supervisors
- Develop cognitive abnormalities (e.g., delusions, hallucinations, and severely disturbed thought processes)

Figure 5.4   Manic Features Not Specified in the DSM-IV(TR)[2, 10]

▲ **Behavioral symptoms**
  ◆ Resistance to treatment
  ◆ Changes in dress, makeup, or appearance to appear more attractive/flamboyant
  ◆ Reckless gambling
  ◆ Antisocial behavior
  ◆ Increased libido
  ◆ Violence
  ◆ Suicide

▲ **Cognitive symptoms**
  ◆ Poor insight
  ◆ Confusion
  ◆ Altered perceptions of smell, hearing, and vision

Clinical Course

In Carlson's and Goodwin's longitudinal study of mood changes in patients with mania, they describe the following three stages of the most classic presentation:[12]

  I. Mood is predominantly euphoric.

  II. Mood becomes irritable, dysphoric, and depressed.

  III. Mood is characterized by anxiety, panic, dysphoria, and psychotic symptoms.

An untreated manic episode usually persists from several weeks to months and may end rather abruptly. While the above describes the classic manifestations, in practice there is a wide range of presentations, including first manic symptoms with a dysphoric mood (dysphoric mania/hypomania).[13]

Characteristics of Mixed Episodes

Both mania and hypomania may contain significant depressive elements. This "mixing" of bipolar phases is rather common. When mania becomes fully mixed with a major depressive episode [a DSM-IV(TR)-defined "Mixed Episode"], the clinical picture is one of agitation and severe irritability with racing thoughts and pressured speech.

> *See chapter four for characteristics of a mixed or "dysphoric" state — a common form of bipolar illness characterized by a mixture of hypomanic and sub-syndromal depressive symptoms.*

Impulsivity and lability of mood can be quite dramatic. Many patients will have suicidal obsessions. Psychotic symptoms may be present and fluctuate in intensity. Indeed, mixed episodes represent situations of heightened risk for suicide, and clinicians should exercise appropriate caution.

Typical features of the mixed episode have been described as related to:[14]

- Dismally low spirits or an emotional state characterized by anxiety, depression, or unease while having a "short-fuse" temper
- Severe agitation
- Anxiety (including panic states) that is resistant to treatment
- Unendurable sexual excitement
- Insomnia that is difficult to remedy or manage
- Suicidal obsessions and impulses
- Genuine expressions of intense suffering while maintaining a melodramatic or "histrionic" demeanor

Diagnostic Criteria for Mixed Episodes

Patients with mixed episodes have symptom duration of at least one week, during which time they meet criteria for both a manic and a major depressive episode. Importantly, the diagnosis is a mixed episode if a patient with mania presents prominent symptoms of a major depressive episode every day for a week or more. (See figure 5.5 below.)

A mixed episode diagnosis does **not** require that the depressive component be present for at least two weeks. Studies indicate that approximately 30 to 40 percent of patients with mania present with mixed symptoms.[15]

Figure 5.5   Criteria for Mixed Episodes[2]

A. The criteria are met both for a Manic Episode (see text) and for a Major Depressive Episode (see text) (except for duration) nearly every day during at least a one-week period.

B. The mood disturbance is sufficiently severe to cause marked impairment in occupational functioning or in usual social activities/relationships with others, or to necessitate hospitalization to prevent harm to self or others; or there are psychotic features.

C. The symptoms are not due to the direct physiological effects of a substance (e.g., a drug of abuse, a medication, or other treatment) or a general medical condition (e.g., hyperthyroidism).

Note: Mixed-like episodes that clearly result from somatic antidepressant treatment (e.g., medication, electroconvulsive therapy, light therapy) should not count toward a diagnosis of bipolar I disorder.

Reprinted with permission of American Psychiatric Association, Diagnostic and Statistical Manual of Mental Disorders, Fourth Edition, Text Revision, Washington, D.C., American Psychiatric Association, 2000.

Clinical manifestations of a mixed episode must be of sufficient magnitude that they produce significant functional impairment or lead to hospitalization and are not secondary to drugs or a general medical condition. The presentation often includes agitation, insomnia, appetite dysregulation, suicide ideation, and psychotic features.

The development of a mixed episode during somatic therapy for depression may be an indication that the patient has a "bipolar diathesis" with an increased risk of later manic, hypomanic, or mixed episodes unrelated to somatic treatments for depression. Debate continues on whether or not development of hypomania during antidepressant treatment indicates a patient will develop bipolar disorders at a later point in time. Ongoing studies should clarify this relationship in the next several years.

Clinical Course

Patients with a mixed episode are more likely to experience depressive delusions and attempt suicide. Failure to recognize the condition can significantly worsen the prognosis.[16-18] Duration of mixed episodes is longer than mania, and relapse may be sooner.

Additionally, differentiation of a mixed episode has significant therapeutic and prognostic implications. If a patient with mixed symptoms is misdiagnosed as having major depression, subsequent antidepressant monotherapy can possibly unmask and exacerbate hypomanic or manic symptoms or induce a manic or hypomanic episode, contributing to treatment resistance for future episodes.[19]

Treating patients with bipolar disorder with antidepressants alone may also result in exacerbated manic/hypomanic symptoms.

References for Chapter 5

1. Suppes T, Mintz, J, McElroy SL, et al. Mixed hypomania in 908 patients with bipolar disorder evaluated prospectively in the Stanley Bipolar Treatment Network: a gender-specific phenomenon. *Archives of General Psychiatry.* 2005 Oct;62:1089–96.

2. American Psychiatric Association, American Psychiatric Association Task Force on DSM-IV. *Diagnostic and Statistical Manual of Mental Disorders: DSM-IV-TR.* Washington, DC; American Psychiatric Association, 2000.

3. Benazzi F, Akiskal HS. Refining the evaluation of bipolar II: beyond the strict SCID-CV guidelines for hypomania. *J Affect Disord.* 2003 Jan;73(1-2):33–8.

4. Judd LL, Akiskal HS, Schettler PJ, et al. A prospective investigation of the natural history of the long-term weekly symptomatic status of bipolar II disorder. *Arch Gen Psychiatry.* 2003 Mar;60(3):261–9.

5. Benazzi F. Is the minimum duration of hypomania in bipolar II disorder 4 days? *Can J Psychiatry.* 2001 Feb;46(1):86.

6. Akiskal HS, Bourgeois ML, Angst J, et al. Re-evaluating the prevalence of and diagnostic composition within the broad clinical spectrum of bipolar disorders. *J Affect Disord.* 2000 Sep;59(Suppl 1):S5 – 30. Review.

7. Benazzi F, Akiskal HS. The duration of hypomania in bipolar-II disorder in private practice: methodology and validation. *J Affect Disord.* 2006;18 (abstracted ahead of publication).

8. Akiskal HS, Maser JD, Zeller PJ, et al. Switching from 'unipolar' to bipolar (II). An 11-year prospective study of clinical and temperamental predictors in 559 patients. *Arch Gen Psychiatry.* 1995 Feb;52(2):114 – 23.

9. Faedda GL, Baldessarini RJ, Suppes T, et al. Pediatric-onset bipolar disorder: a neglected clinical and public health problem. *Harv Rev Psychiatry.* 1995;3(4):171 – 95.

10. Keck PE Jr, McElroy SL, Arnold LM. Bipolar disorder. *Med Clin North Am.* 2001;85(3):645 – 61, ix.Review

11. American Psychiatric Association. Practice guideline for the treatment of patients with bipolar disorder (revision). *Am J Psychiatry.* 2002;159(4 Suppl):1 – 50.

12. Carlson GA, Goodwin FK. The stages of mania. A longitudinal analysis of the manic episode. *Arch Gen Psychiatry.* 1973;28(2):221 – 8.

13. Goodwin FK, Jamison KR. *Manic-Depressive Illness.* New York, NY: Oxford University Press; 1990.

14. Akiskal HS, Mallya G. Criteria for the "soft" bipolar spectrum – treatment implications. *Psychopharmacology Bulletin.* 1987;23(1):68 – 73.

15. McElroy SL, Keck PE Jr, Pope HG Jr, et al. Clinical and research implications of the diagnosis of dysphoric or mixed mania or hypomania. *Am J Psychiatry.* 1992;149(12):1633 – 44.

16. Dilsaver SC, Chen YW, Swann AC, et al. Suicidality in patients with pure and depressive mania. *Am J Psychiatry* 1994;151(9):1312 – 5.

17. Strakowski SM, McElroy SL, Keck PE Jr, West SA. Suicidality among patients with mixed and manic bipolar disorder. *Am J Psychiatry.* 1996; 153(5):674 – 6.

18. Strakowski SM, Tohen M, Stoll A. Comorbidity in mania at first hospitalization. *Am J Psychiatry.* 1992;149:554 – 6.

19. Kupfer DJ, Carpenter LL, Frank E. Possible role of antidepressants in precipitating mania and hypomania in recurrent depression. *Am J Psychiatry.* 1988;145(7):804 – 8.

Chapter 6:
Assess for Distress/Dysfunction

Primary care clinicians are well positioned to assess and diagnose bipolar illness due to a number of factors:

- The family history may be more readily available, and bipolar illness' strong heritability demands a careful examination of that history.

- There may be more of a lifelong perspective of health care that makes the longitudinal trajectory of the illness, beginning with its roots in temperament, apparent at an early age.

  Informed and interested clinicians, accurately assessing the bipolar illness diathesis, can be alert to temperament and monitor for early-onset syndromal episodes.

  This is especially true when one's practice includes multi-generational families.

- Pragmatically speaking, patients with mental distress and dysfunction often present first in the primary care setting. The usual presentation is somatic. Depressed and anxious patients must be screened closely for bipolar disorder.

- The existing therapeutic alliance may improve communication, particularly regarding the illness' existential qualities.

Recent data on medical comorbidity also suggests that primary care physicians can contribute to a comprehensive treatment approach. For example, it is now known that obesity, metabolic syndrome, and perhaps type II diabetes mellitus (T2DM) are more common in those with bipolar illness, and that treatments for bipolar disorder can affect both metabolic and lipid parameters.[1-3]

This chapter covers information-gathering strategies for assessing the level of a patient's distress and/or dysfunction, including:

- Conducting the initial interview
- Assessing psychiatric history
- Assessing family history
- Assessing medical history/laboratory findings

The last section of the chapter presents a time-management approach that incorporates these strategies and the use of validated screening tools in the typical primary care practitioner's available schedule. Although referred to as part of the clinical process throughout this chapter, detailed information on assessment measures used in both primary care and psychiatric settings appears in chapter 15.

> **Note:** Results from validated screening tools are **not** necessarily indicative of the presence of bipolar disorder.[4]

Conducting the Initial Interview

In the course of the initial interview, it can be helpful to first ask questions in an open-ended fashion so that the physician has the opportunity to determine the basis for the visit.

Patients exhibiting mental distress typically present to primary care with somatic complaints.[5] For bipolar patients experiencing symptoms, this more often occurs during times of significant depression.[6] At these times, fatigue, headache, gastrointestinal dysfunction, sleep abnormalities, and pain are common.

> See pages 81 through 92 later in this chapter for an approach to initial interviewing that maximizes time spent with the patient in 15- to 20-minute segments.

Clinicians should inquire about mood, anxiety, and substance use in all such patients, especially when complaints are chronic and when alternate explanations are not readily found. These patients may also be diagnosed with:

- Irritable bowel syndrome
- Non-ulcer dyspepsia
- Migraine or chronic daily headache
- Chronic fatigue syndrome

Evaluating how symptoms impact a patient's ability to function at work, home, or in avocational endeavors is also appropriate.

Patients presenting first to the mental health system are more likely to have severe or life-threatening symptoms, or to have self-selected that sector based on insight, support systems, reduced financial barriers, or other factors. Many patients are seen initially in primary care, making assessment (even assessment of need for referral) a critical function of that care.

As the interview progresses, questions may become more focused to obtain specific information, such as dates of symptom onset and duration of episodes. Since patients with psychiatric illnesses may not always be the best historians, a definite diagnosis of bipolar disorder cannot always be made from patient self-report. In fact, lack of insight is often a component of bipolar disorder. Therefore, it is often important to elicit supplemental and corroborating information from the patient's family members, significant others, and associates.

Using Established Mnemonics for Evaluating Symptoms

Those with bipolar disorder often present as depressed. Less often, they present with mixed or dysphoric hypomania (co-occurring depressive manifestations with hypomania), or mania. The following describes two mnemonics — DIGFAST and SAD-A-FACES — typically used to help evaluate symptoms presented.

DIGFAST and the Patient with Mania

The seven "B" criteria (listed in figure 5.3 on page 58 in chapter 5) for the diagnosis of mania/hypomania can be recalled by the mnemonic DIGFAST. (See figure 6.1 on the next page.)[7] A manic/hypomanic disorder is present if three (if euphoric) or four (if irritable) DIGFAST criteria are present.

With mania, unlike hypomania, significant dysfunction exists in the social and/or occupational domain. Thus, a patient with the appropriate number of DIGFAST criteria who is neither impaired nor psychotic, or who does not require hospitalization, is likely experiencing a hypomanic episode. Furthermore, manic symptoms must be present for at least one week (unless hospitalization is necessary), while hypomania can be diagnosed after only four days of DIGFAST symptoms. Hypomania with psychotic features automatically is defined as a manic episode. Patients with mixed or dysphoric hypomania should be coded as having hypomania, regardless of associated mood symptoms.

Chapter 5 presents information on initial presentation of mania/ hypomania; chapter 8 lists DSM-IV(TR) criteria for diagnosis.

Figure 6.1 DIGFAST Mnemonic For Mania/Hypomania[4]

- **DISTRACTIBILITY:** Inability to maintain one's focus on tasks for an extended duration

- **INSOMNIA:** Decreased need for sleep coupled with increased energy in manic/hypomanic patients (must be differentiated from the insomnia of major depressive episode)

- **GRANDIOSITY:** Unrealistic, high self-confidence or delusional

- **FLIGHT OF IDEAS:** Racing thoughts

- **ACTIVITIES:** Increased goal-directed activities that may be appropriate in their nature, but clearly excessive, occurring in social, sexual, school, or workplace domains

- **SPEECH:** Significantly more talkative compared to periods of euthymia

- **THOUGHTLESSNESS:** Dysfunctional, self-centered activities, such as: spending sprees, unprotected sex with strangers, and other impulsive behaviors

INTRODUCTION

PRESENTATION

CLINICAL PROCESS

PHARMACOTHERAPY

RESOURCES

SAD-A-FACES and the Patient with Depression

A bipolar disorder diagnosis should be considered for any patient presenting with symptoms of a major depressive episode. Criteria for a major depressive episode can be recalled with the mnemonic SAD-A-FACES as shown in figure 6.2 below.[8]

Figure 6.2   SAD-A-FACES Mnemonic for Depression[8]

SAD

- **SLEEP** disturbance (insomnia/hypersomnia)
- **APPETITE** or weight change
- **DYSPHORIA** "bad mood"

-A-

- **ANHEDONIA**

FACES

- **FATIGUE**
- **AGITATION**/motor retardation
- **CONCENTRATION** diminished
- **ESTEEM** (low)/guilt
- **SUICIDE**/thoughts of death

A single manic or hypomanic episode changes a diagnosis from one of major depressive episode to bipolar disorder, most recent episode depressed. See chapter 4 for information on initial presentation of depression; see chapter 7 for differential diagnostic information related to unipolar vs. bipolar depression. Chapter 8 lists relevant DSM-IV(TR) criteria for diagnosis.

Assessing Psychiatric History

A major goal in examining the psychiatric history of patients with possible bipolar disorder is to determine if they have had at least one manic or hypomanic episode at some time in their lives.

The history of the present illness should include a chronology of events related to the chief complaint, including recent exacerbations, remissions, and responses to therapeutic interventions. It is helpful to ask if changes in mood have affected the patient's life at home, work, or school. For example, has periodic irritability impacted work and/or home environment and relationships?

Establishing age of onset of symptoms is particularly important. The National Depressive and Manic-Depressive Association (NDMDA), which is now the Depression and Bipolar Support Alliance (DBSA), conducted a survey of their members in 1994. In that survey, the peak period of onset was identified as between 15 and 19 years old, and first symptoms were reported during childhood for 31 percent of the respondents.[9] The study was conducted again in 2000 with 33 percent of respondents reporting being under age 15 when symptoms first appeared.[10] The percentage of those reporting onset at the 15- to 19-year period was 27 percent in that later study.

The presence of any past psychiatric episodes or care may provide a clue to the diagnosis. Since patients with bipolar disorder may have previously been treated with antidepressants, the following clues will help the physician identify bipolar disorder in patients treated with antidepressants:

- "Refractory depression," an initial rapid response followed by increasing drug-resistance
- Illness course worsened by antidepressant therapy

INTRODUCTION

PRESENTATION

CLINICAL PROCESS

PHARMACOTHERAPY

RESOURCES

> *Patients with a rapid cycling course comprise approximately 10 to 20 percent of the overall population of patients with bipolar disorder.[4]*

- Rapid mood swings (cycling) in response to medication
- The need for combination therapy with an antidepressant plus a mood stabilizer such as lithium

Patients with bipolar disorder are more likely than the general population to have problems with the legal system. Inquiries should be made about arrests (including driving under the influence), jail time, probation, upcoming court dates, etc. Additionally, the use of alcohol and substances should be carefully explored given the high lifetime prevalence of alcohol and substance use disorders in patients with bipolar disorder.

> *Abuse of some drugs, including cocaine and corticosteroids, can cause bipolar-like syndromes. (See chapter 7 for more information on substance abuse and differential diagnosis.)*

Psychoactive substances can induce secondary mood disorders. The presence of substance use disorder does not rule out a diagnosis of mood disorder. However, if episodes of abnormal mood exclusively develop during episodes of substance abuse, the diagnosis changes to substance-induced mood disorder. Substance-induced mood disorder must be differentiated from the use of substances to ameliorate affective symptoms (see chapter 7 for information on substance abuse, differential diagnosis, and comorbidity). A careful medication history must also be taken (e.g., both corticosteroids and L-Dopa can induce secondary mania).

JANICE

Clinician: *"How old were you when you had your first experience with depression?"*

Janice: *"I never really experienced depression until the last year. I'm typically an outgoing, energetic person with a tendency to act impulsively and get in trouble."* (This was her explanation for a DUI conviction and a "Las Vegas" wedding that ended in divorce in less than six months.) *"Mostly, I'm a wonderful, loving, kind-hearted person — really!"*

Clinician: *"What treatment have you had in the past?"*

Janice: *"I've only had specific treatment twice: once when I briefly sought help from a psychotherapist after my divorce and the other when I had to go to court-ordered counseling after the DUI."*

From this line of questioning, the clinician determines that Janice has predominately manic symptoms in the form of hypomanic and a likely manic episode (Vegas wedding) prior to her first depression, which was in the form of a mixed state. No medical treatment had ever been prescribed for her mood disturbances. In fact, the clinician senses that Janice's "mistakes" were counted as problems of personality or temperament and not ascribed to an axis I disorder such as bipolar illness.

BILL

Clinician: *"How old were you when you had your first significant experience with depression?"*

Bill: *"I remember one- to two-day periods of intense sadness as early as age seven. I wandered through the woods behind my house crying for no reason. These episodes lasted throughout adolescence and occasionally as long as two to four weeks. But I don't remember ever going to a doctor or getting any treatment for it."*

When Bill recounted that he had never received treatment for these episodes, the clinician began to probe for evidence of mania.

Clinician: *"Do you have days of energy or increased activity that come and go abruptly? Have you ever experienced a period of persistently or distinctly increased energy?"*

Bill: *"I remember long, fairly intense periods of great energy and activity that began during college. I felt unstoppable and brilliant. I could go days or weeks with little or no sleep. At times though, rage was a real problem. I was arrested for assault on one occasion. I also did a lot of drinking during that time. However, that kind of energy is a rare thing these days!"*

INTRODUCTION

PRESENTATION

CLINICAL PROCESS

PHARMACOTHERAPY

RESOURCES

Bill's account of his college experiences tells the clinician that there is likely a history of manic episodes preceding the current depression.

Assessing Family History

Because bipolar disorder has a strong genetic basis, it is important to question the patient about a family history of mood disorders. This should include focused questions about the presence of specific hypomanic, manic, or depressive symptoms in family members — particularly first-degree relatives. Other clues may be suicide attempts or hospitalizations for mental illness. Where a history of suicide exists for family members, the patient can have a higher suicide risk.

Family history assessment should also determine the presence of psychiatric comorbidities associated with bipolar disorder and the use of mental health medications by family members. For example, a relative may have been identified as alcoholic and having problems with anger vs. being identified as having bipolar disorder and substance abuse. A social history must also be included as it may reveal changes in interpersonal relationships that result from bipolar symptoms or interpersonal difficulties secondary to a comorbidity commonly associated with bipolar disorder.

> *Patients with first-degree relatives with established diagnoses of bipolar disorder are at higher risk for bipolar disorder themselves.*

JANICE

Clinician: *"Do problems like depression or anxiety or substance abuse run in your family?"*

Janice: *"I have a brother diagnosed with bipolar disorder. My mother had frequent problems with really bad depressions; once she had to be in a psychiatric hospital for awhile. My grandfather (maternal) was moody and brilliant, an accomplished jazz pianist … and a hopeless alcoholic."*

Janice's genogram (with family members described as having mood disorders numbered) appears below.

Figure 6.3   Genogram for Janice

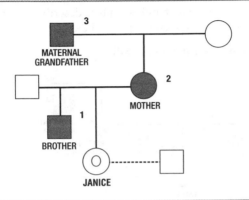

BILL

Clinician: *"Do problems like depression or anxiety or substance abuse run in your family?"*

Bill: *"My father was an alcoholic with severe mood swings; his brother and sisters were always depressed and one was even institutionalized at one point. My grandmother (paternal) was an eccentric woman from a very angry family. Way back, her brother murdered four men in a bar room brawl and was known to shoot at the houses of those with whom he was 'feuding'. My two sons and daughter have had various problems with using drugs and alcohol as well as sometimes being impulsive and violent."*

Clinician: *"You mentioned the tragic death of your daughter. How did that happen?"*

Bill: *"She was drunk, walking on the side of the road, and walked into the path of a car. That was nearly four years ago."*

His daughter's death is the event that appears to have triggered Bill's most recent episode of depression. What can be

INTRODUCTION

PRESENTATION

CLINICAL PROCESS

PHARMACOTHERAPY

RESOURCES

gleaned from his answers is the presence of impairing mood disorder in three consecutive generations with behavior that can be easily connected to periods of persistent irritable mood with marked impairment in behavior or function.

Bill's genogram (with family members described as having mood disorders numbered) appears below.

Figure 6.4   Genogram for Bill

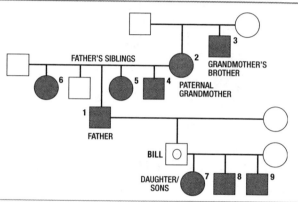

Assessing Medical History/Laboratory Findings

A patient's history should rule out the possibility that the symptoms result from use of a substance or medication, or from a general medical disorder.

Important measures to obtain for ruling out a primary medical cause for mania include:

- Baseline complete blood count (CBC)
- Thyroid hormone assay (TSH, T3, and T4)
- Fasting glucose and lipid profile (total cholesterol and HDL-C)

Refer to chapter 7 for detailed differential diagnostic information.

- Hepatic function tests (transaminase levels)
- Renal function test (creatinine and BUN)

Past history of head injury should always be part of a medical assessment for the possibility of bipolar disorder because head injury in and of itself can be either a causal or an aggravating factor for bipolar symptoms. Given that many untreated patients with bipolar disorder have low impulse control and a tendency to engage in risky behavior, the possibility for head injury becomes particularly pertinent. In general, physicians should consider a brain scan for those patients who have never had one.

Laboratory Findings and Mania

There are no laboratory tests for diagnosing mania. However, a variety of abnormal laboratory findings have been identified in patients with manic episodes, including abnormalities of sleep physiology, dysregulation of the hypothalamic-pituitary-adrenal axis, and dysregulation of neurotransmission and neuroendocrine activity.[11] These physiological changes are not used for diagnostic purposes; they are indicative of the manic state, studied in an effort to further our understanding of the biologic basis of bipolar disorder.

Laboratory findings to pinpoint other causes of manic symptoms are important as symptoms can result from substance abuse (e.g., psychostimulants) and general medical conditions (e.g., hyperthyroidism).

New onset mania in later life is particularly associated with secondary causes and high rates of neurological and medical illnesses. Right hemispheric brain lesions are especially common among neurological causes.

Laboratory Findings and Depression

As many as 90 percent of patients with major depression will have abnormal sleep physiology.[11] Polysomnography may show manifestations described above plus:

- Abnormal rapid eye movement (REM)
- Shifts in non-REM activity away from a first sleep period
- Increased duration of REM early in sleep

There are a variety of neuroendocrine abnormalities associated with major depression. These include abnormalities of the major neurotransmitter systems as well as disordered hypothalamic-pituitary-adrenal axis (HPAA) physiology (e.g., increased urinary free cortisol levels, failure of dexamethasone to suppress cortisol secretion). In addition, other hormones whose secretory amounts and patterns rely on the hypothalamus and pituitary may have blunted responses to various provocative tests. Functional brain imaging studies during major depressive episodes demonstrate shifts in cortical blood flow and metabolism from the lateral prefrontal cortex to the limbic and paralimbic regions.

Laboratory Findings and Mixed Episodes

There are no laboratory findings for diagnosing mixed episodes. Of note are the findings of dysregulation of the hypothalmic-pituitary-adrenal axis, neurotransmitters, and neuroendocrine system that show elements of manic and depressive changes.[11]

Interviewing Those Close to the Patient

Lack of insight is a common problem in bipolar disorder, resulting in patients sometimes consciously minimizing symptoms or failing to accurately see themselves within their psychosocial surroundings. Denial is an often-used defense when grandiosity is present. An amplification of natural tendencies to blame others may be present as well. In the case of hypomania, a change in behavior observable by others is a necessary component of the diagnosis.

In the replicated NDMDA (now DBSA) study, published in 2003, patients significantly under-reported manic symptoms of heightened mood (40 percent) and increased activity (38 percent).[10] However, most respondents reported depressive symptoms, which can mean a greater potential for misdiagnosis.[10] Accordingly, including significant others in patient assessment is often critical.[12–14] Establishing such a relationship will also be important when tracking treatment response. Even if a diagnosis of major depressive disorder is made, clinicians will want to occasionally interview those close to the patient for potential signs of emerging mania/hypomania.[15]

One way to transition to interviewing important others in the patient's life might be to ask how their symptoms are affecting those close to them (e.g., family, co-workers). After opening the subject in this way, a follow-up question might ask for, even emphasize, the participation of a significant other to provide important information relating to diagnosis and treatment planning. Follow-up visits might be planned specifically to include significant others.

In situations of severe illness, the patient may be accompanied by a concerned other or even be compelled by such individuals to seek care. It may be useful to give duplicate screening tools, such as the Mood Disorder Questionnaire, to the significant other and ask that they endorse the symptoms of mania and level of impairment that they have observed in the patient as a way of corroborating and elucidating symptoms and the circumstances driving treat-

For information on the Mood Disorder Questionnaire, see pages 284 through 285 in chapter 15.

ment. The separately completed documents may then be compared for discrepancies in an open discussion.

Suicide and Homicide Risk

Patients with bipolar disorder have 10 to 15 percent lifetime suicide rates.[14] Every patient who may have bipolar disorder or describes depressive symptoms should be asked about suicidal ideation, plans or preparations for suicide, and intent to act on those plans. They should also be asked about access to medications or firearms that may be used to commit suicide. In most instances, suicide attempts are associated with depressive manifestations, either during a major depressive or mixed episode.

INTRODUCTION PRESENTATION CLINICAL PROCESS PHARMACOTHERAPY RESOURCES

The potential suicide risk factors for those with bipolar disorder include:[16, 17]

- Early age of onset
- Numerous depressive episodes
- Comorbid alcohol abuse
- Personal history of antidepressant-induced mania
- Family history of suicidal behavior
- Impulsivity and hostility

Additionally, patients with bipolar disorder, who do attempt suicide, typically choose more violent, lethal means than those suffering unipolar depression. In one study of 2,395 psychiatric inpatients, patients with bipolar disorder were six times more likely to select highly lethal methods for attempting suicide, which suggests potentially more completed suicides.[18]

JANICE

When Janice talks about having trouble sleeping, she describes a strategy she uses for getting to sleep where she fantasizes that someone is drilling a hole in her head to let all of the "excess thoughts" out. Janice also reports feeling increasingly trapped and hopeless. She spends a lot of time thinking about driving her car into a bridge abutment. She had considered purchasing a gun.

Because hopelessness is an important feature of suicidality and she has actively considered a lethal means, the clinician makes arrangements for immediate referral to a psychiatrist and close coordination with psychiatric and/or hospital staff.

While homicidal behavior is uncommon, clinicians should also query a patient as to aggressive impulses towards others. A past history of aggressive behavior or legal difficulties (as well as aggressive behavior associated with alcohol or other substance use) should be explored.

Time Management in Primary Care Environment

Practically speaking, primary care physicians rarely have 60 consecutive minutes available to spend with a patient; however, various approaches can give the clinician the same outcomes, especially those that combine time management principles and brief psychotherapy strategies, such as those outlined in the book, *The Fifteen-Minute Hour*.[19] These psychotherapy strategies are compatible with the typical office visit; one published strategy uses the acronym BATHE shown in figure 6.5 below.

Figure 6.5   BATHE Psychotherapy Strategy
(adapted from Lieberman & Stuart, 1999)[20]

BATHE Acronym Components	Target Information
BACKGROUND — "What is going on in your life?"	To elicit the context of the visit
AFFECT — "How do you feel about that?"	To ascertain emotional response to the context
TROUBLE — "What troubles you the most about this situation?"	To assess symbolic meaning of context
HANDLING — "How are you handling that?"	To determine patient's responses and available resources
EMPATHY — "That must be very difficult for you."	To acknowledge response as appropriate to situation

For most patients seen in the primary care setting, using three or four, 15- to 20-minute increments can be very productive for information gathering. Coordinating the initial assessment process (interview, patient completion of self-report instruments, patient education,

Do not use the BATHE method if the patient is resistant, hostile, or presents psychotic symptoms or is in severe pain or suffering life-threatening circumstances. For domestic violence or other abuse, further inquiry and possible action is mandatory.

and lab/x-ray testing) around seeing several patients within a one- to two-hour period can be an effective way to spend needed time with those suffering from psychiatric as well as medical conditions. For example, a clinician can spend 15 to 20 minutes with a new patient exhibiting symptoms of a mood disturbance, then leave the patient alone with material to read and complete, see another patient, and come back and spend five more minutes getting additional information. Next, someone from the lab can come in while the clinician sees a third patient. The clinician then comes back into the room to discuss treatment approach/additional tests. The following presents three of these "segments:"

Segment One: Targeting Possible Mood Disorder

This process builds on whatever chief complaint the patient presents — if the chief complaint looks like a somatic problem that is chronic and refractory and the patient has multiple problems on their list, the clinician might ask initial questions, such as:

- Have you recently had difficulty with depressed mood or lack of interest in your usual activities?
- Have you had difficulty with insomnia or irritability?

If the responses are positive, the clinician would want to test for possible anxiety disorder by asking:

- Do you seem to have problems with excessive worry?

At this point, the clinician might say, "I need to get a little more information about what's going on with you. Here are some questions I'd like you to respond to while I'm out of the room. If you finish before I get back, there are also some information sheets you might want to read over." The clinician then leaves the patient with a packet that contains a copy of some well-validated, self-report assessment tools, such as:

- **The PHQ-9 (Patient Health Questionnaire)** — A depression screening tool
- **The MDQ (Mood Disorder Questionnaire) and**

BSDS (Bipolar Spectrum Diagnostic Scale) — Bipolar disorder screening tools

See chapter 15 for detailed information on the PHQ-9, MDQ, BSDS, the TEMPS-A, and other validated assessment scales. **Note:** *Results from screening tools are* **not** *necessarily indicative of illness.*

• **The TEMPS-A (Temperament Evaluation of Memphis, Pisa, Paris and San Diego Autoquestionnaire version)** — A temperament profile

The packet also contains patient information, such as handouts on depression/anxiety and bipolar disorder.

Besides the assessment tools mentioned in this process (PHQ-9, MDQ, BSDS, and TEMPS-A), various psychometric instruments are reviewed in chapter 15 (section E). These types of tools, although typically not part of primary care practice, can be used to enhance one's knowledge of bipolar illness. For example, the Young Mania Rating Scale (YMRS) allows primary care physicians to learn how to talk about mania and what to ask patients to elicit diagnostic clues.

It is important for the clinician to briefly describe why they've asked the patient to complete these forms as well as to ensure they understand how to fill out the questionnaires. If a family member or friend has accompanied the patient, they should be invited to read the handouts while the patient completes the questionnaires. Ask the patient to see if something in the handout feels like it might apply to them.

Segment Two: Targeting Family/Psychiatric History

In about 20 minutes, the clinician returns to the room and reviews the materials, asking the patient for feedback ("How do you feel about all this?"). Then, using the results of the questionnaires, the clinician probes for additional information. If there are positive responses on the questionnaires, one might ask questions, such as those in figure 6.6 on the following page.

INTRODUCTION

PRESENTATION

CLINICAL PROCESS

PHARMACOTHERAPY

RESOURCES

Figure 6.6   Family/Psychiatric History Interviewing

Interview Question	Target Information/ Special Concerns
How old were you when you had your first significant episode of depression?	Depression beginning in childhood or adolescence significantly raises the possibility of bipolar illness.
How long did it last? How severe was it? Did you notice that your sleep was disturbed, that you had significant problems functioning in school or in other places in your life?	It is important to verify the presence of significant impairment for past depressive symptoms.
What treatment did you receive for that depression? How did you respond to the treatment? Have antidepressants ever made you worse? More depressed? More agitated? Did the medications stop working after several weeks or months?	Lack of response or treatment-emergent manic symptomatology treatment response may be indicative of bipolar illness.
How many episodes do you think you have had since that first episode? Is depression a constant or an episodic part of your life?	These questions are important differentiating major depression, dysthymic disorder, and bipolar disorder.
Does psychiatric illness run in your family, specifically depression, bipolar disorder, manic-depression, anxiety, alcoholism, or other substance abuse? Do family members seem to have difficulty controlling their emotions?	Bipolar disorder is more likely among those with: • A first-degree relative with bipolar disorder • Three+ first-degree relatives with impairing mood disorders • Three consecutive generations with impairing mood disorders

At this point in the interview, the clinician could begin drawing a genogram based on the patient's answers — a process that takes another five minutes or so. A genogram is quite valuable because it displays the structure of intergenerational relationships in addition to psychosocial and health status information. Having this visual display of the complexities of family relationships and, often, prevalence of psychiatric illness can be a valuable tool for validating and communicating the genetic qualities of bipolar illness.

Asking the patient about their psychiatric history targets information needed to make a differential diagnosis (see chapter 7). Having a positive family history of depression is not necessarily indicative of possible bipolar illness; however, the likelihood of a relationship between the two is great. The family histories most fraught with psychiatric illness are likely to reveal more bipolar than unipolar illness.

Segment Three: Targeting Hypomania

Additional questioning can target symptoms of hypomania that may go undiagnosed or misdiagnosed as major depression. Questions could include:

- When was the last time you felt normal or had significant energy? Tell me what that looked like?
- Did you notice that you needed less sleep?
- How long did this period of increased energy last? Have you ever noticed that such a period lasted several days?
- During that time, did you feel you needed less sleep at night?
- Did your mind seem to be overly active?
- Did you have a sense that your thoughts were racing?
- Did you feel like your thoughts were stuffed into your head; you had too much to think about; and it was all passing by too fast for you to sort through?
- Were you cleaning and rearranging furniture in the early morning hours?

INTRODUCTION

PRESENTATION

CLINICAL PROCESS

PHARMACOTHERAPY

RESOURCES

- Did you make plans for the future that either you couldn't get done or lost interest in after the passion and energy wore off?

- Did you do things during that period that you later regretted?

- Were you optimistic vs. being pessimistic?

- Did you feel elated or have a sense of unrestrained self-importance, or did you feel much more irritable than usual?

Segment Four: Targeting Next Steps

Using this approach, 10–15 minutes of a clinician's face-to-face time with the patient can result in having a pretty good sense of whether the patient's treatment needs fall within the clinician's scope of practice or would be better met by a psychiatrist. For example, strong, positive responses to questions about early onset and family history as well as a PHQ-9 in the severe range and a positive MDQ are reasonable indications that a physician is probably dealing with a patient with bipolar illness, and most likely bipolar II disorder. The clinician can then make treatment decisions based on how much they know about bipolar disorder, their comfort level with making such a diagnosis, whether or not the patient may be a danger to themselves or others, and what their current knowledge base is regarding treatment approaches and side-effect management.

Depending on the information gathered, the patient's risk of harming themselves or others, and medical history, the clinician may want to schedule a follow up appointment or have the patient return later in the day following additional testing (e.g., lab work, x-rays, CT scan). Additionally, the clinician may want to consult with a colleague on the case before moving forward with treatment or referral. The patient's response (and those of family members/friends) may indicate that the patient needs a day or two to process new information (appropriate **only** if symptoms are not severe or life-threatening).

Thus, in the initial interview, the clinician is putting together pieces of the puzzle — family history of psychiatric illness, early onset of illness (typically more depressive in nature), not responding to antidepressant treatment (either no response or treatment-triggered hypomanic/manic episodes/symptoms) — until a picture emerges that is more likely to be bipolar disorder.

> *It is important to remember that although indicative of possible bipolar illness, earlier onset and family history are not absolutes. Clinicians should consider the diagnosis of bipolar illness before treating other conditions, especially depression. In cases where the diagnosis is in doubt, consultation is recommended.*

To illustrate how this process might work with a specific patient, the following examines information gathered with Holly, the case study patient who appears to be suffering from hypomania. Note that evidence exists that a clinical interview sensitive for the detection of hypomania should focus initially on the psychomotor activation and associated behaviors followed by confirmation of the abnormally elevated, expansive, depressed, or irritable mood. This investigation supports earlier investigations of outpatients in that bipolar II is differentiated from unipolar major depression by an earlier age of onset, trait mood lability, higher rates of depressive recurrences, higher rates of atypical features, hypomanic symptoms during depressive episodes, and greater familial loading for bipolar disorders.[21]

HOLLY

Holly's chief reason for seeing her primary care physician today is a migraine headache. Note that migraine headache is common in patients (especially women) suffering from bipolar disorder.[22] Her clinician recounts the initial visit:

> **Clinician**: *"When I walked into the room, I noticed very quickly that this patient appeared depressed. As I asked questions about depressed or anxious moods, my eyes and ears were in agreement – this was a sad lady having problems with depression but presenting with headache."*

INTRODUCTION

PRESENTATION

CLINICAL PROCESS

PHARMACOTHERAPY

RESOURCES

Segment One:
Targeting Holly's Possible Mood Disorder

Clinician: *"Are you having problems with feeling sad or depressed?"*

Holly: *"You would be depressed too if you had this headache."*

The clinician was not particularly swayed by this last comment because it was indicative of the pain of the moment and, perhaps, some level of irritability and grandiosity that may extend into other areas.

The clinician then reported:

"I had in the corner of my eye the husband, who was shaking his head as if to say, 'Oh boy, does she have problems with depression.' Her husband was there to drive her home because they were expecting a shot for pain."

"I knew very quickly that I needed to get additional information and having her complete self-report questionnaires was part of the alliance-building process. I wanted her to show interest. A key element in patient care is having a person take a role in their own diagnosis and treatment. By taking more time to complete and review these questionnaires and talk, I demonstrated to her that I was interested — she's used to being treated for her migraines by getting a shot and being sent home as quickly as possible. The idea that I would extend the time to ask about this level of detail was highly unusual in her experience. It told her that I wanted to know more and that meant that I was interested in her."

Later, when asked about the days of energy that come and go abruptly, Holly's husband confirmed that this was the case and that the quality of those energetic periods was very often irritable.

Holly's Husband: *"I just know to get out of the way. It doesn't matter if I try to confront her or console her — there is nothing good that I can do and no positive gesture that would not be subject to misinterpretation."*

Holly completes a PHQ-9 and an MDQ; she and her husband review the patient information materials provided.

Segment Two:
Targeting Holly's Family/Psychiatric History

After about 20 minutes, the clinician returned to the room and asked about family and psychiatric history.

> **Clinician:** *"Do problems like depression or anxiety or substance abuse run in your family?"*

> **Holly:** *"Oh, yes! You probably don't have time to hear about my family. My father was the proverbial 'rolling stone.' He was a violent alcoholic who either married or shacked up with a number of women. His brother committed suicide, and their father was a severe alcoholic. My sister has made several suicide attempts."*

Holly's genogram (with family members described as having mood disorders numbered) appears below.

Figure 6.7   Genogram for Holly

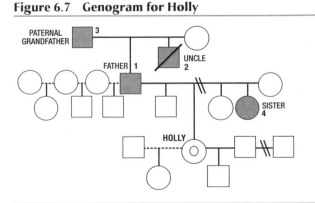

> **Clinician:** *"How old were you when you had your first significant experience with depression?"*

> **Holly:** *"I overdosed on pain pills when I was 13. I can remember being depressed even before that. I've always been moody and, to be honest, a bit of a 'drama queen.'"*

> **Clinician:** *"Have you ever been treated for depression?"*

INTRODUCTION · PRESENTATION · CLINICAL PROCESS · PHARMACOTHERAPY · RESOURCES

Holly: *"Many times. I've been treated with five or six antidepressants and had combinations of several. Mostly they haven't worked at all or made me worse – sometimes I felt like I was "on speed." Sertraline seemed like a miracle for about three weeks; then it stopped working."*

Segment Three: Targeting Holly's Hypomania

Clinician: *"Do you have days of energy or increased activity that come and go abruptly?"*

Holly: *"I can sometimes go through periods – for a few days or a week or so – when everything is easy. I have a lot of energy and get lots of things done. I feel restless. I started back to school to get an associates degree in accounting during a time like that. But the energy never lasts. I lose interest and quit whatever I'm doing."*

Clinician: *"Is your sleep different during these periods of energy? Do you feel as if your thoughts are speeded up or racing or crowded?"*

Holly: *"I need less sleep. Maybe only three hours. My mind moves so fast I can hardly keep up with thoughts. It makes it very hard to concentrate."*

Clinician: *"What is your mood like during these periods of energy?"*

Holly: *"I'm occasionally happy during those times, but usually I'm angry. My family avoids me. My husband says it's like a storm that passes after a few days."*

Holly appeared to be describing a one-week period of distinctly irritable or elated mood accompanied by increased activity, decreased need for sleep, racing thoughts, and distractibility that met the DSM-IV(TR) criteria for hypomania. Given Holly's family history and the impact of her "hypomania" on her family, consideration was also given to the possibility of bipolar I disorder.

To conduct a more detailed evaluation, the clinician reviewed presenting symptoms as well as her answers to assessment questions to see if there were some "matches" or contradictions that needed to be explored.

HOLLY'S PHQ-9 AND CLINICIAN COMMENTARY

Over the last 2 weeks, how often have you been bothered by any of the following problems?	Not at all	Several days	More than half the days	Nearly every day
1.) Little interest or pleasure in doing things	0	1	2	③
2.) Feeling down, depressed, or hopeless	0	1	②	3
3.) Trouble falling or staying asleep, or sleeping too much	0	1	②	3
4.) Feeling tired or having little energy	0	1	②	3
5.) Poor appetite or overeating	0	①	2	3
6.) Feeling bad about yourself–that you are a failure or have let yourself or your family down	0	①	2	3
7.) Trouble concentrating on things, such as reading the newspaper or watching television	0	①	2	3
8.) Moving or speaking so slowly that other people could have noticed? Or the opposite–being so fidgety or restless that you have been moving around a lot more than usual	0	①	2	3
9.) Thoughts that you would be better off dead or hurting yourself in some way	╱0	①	2	3
(For office coding: Total Score)		5	6	3
If you have experienced any of these problems, how difficult have they made it for you to do your work, take care of things at home, or get along with other people?				
☐ Not difficult at all	☐ Somewhat difficult	☒ Very difficult	☐ Extremely difficult	

PHQ-9 Copyright ©1999 Pfizer Inc. All rights reserved. Reproduced with permission.

Clinician: *"Holly's PHQ looked better than she did. Maybe the headache made her look worse. Anything above an 11 on the total score roughly correlates with major depressive disorder. In terms of general scoring, she doesn't quite catch a full-blown depression because of lines 1 and 2. Her score does roughly correlate with major depressive disorder. This tells me that decreased motivation is the most prominent symptom. I always look at item #9 for suicidality; you need to act quickly if passive or active thoughts emerge. Documenting what current depression looks like, knowing it's recurrent from history, and that there are hypomanic episodes in just the last two weeks tends to make me think it is not unipolar depression."*

HOLLY'S MDQ AND CLINICIAN COMMENTARY

Has there ever been a period of time when you were not your usual self and...	YES	NO
...you felt so good or so hyper that other people thought that you were not your normal self or you were so hyper that you got into trouble?	✗	
...you were so irritable that you shouted at people or started fights or arguments?	✗	
...you felt much more self-confident than usual?		✗
...you got much less sleep than usual and found you didn't really miss it?	✗	
...you were much more talkative and/or spoke much faster than usual?		✗
...thoughts raced through your head and/or your couldn't slow your mind down?	✗	
...you were so easily distracted by things around you that you had trouble concentrating or staying on track?		✗
...you had much more energy than usual?		✗
...you were much more active and/or did many more things than usual?		✗
...you were much more social or outgoing than usual–for example, you telephoned friends in the middle of the night?	✗	
...you were much more interested in sex than usual?		✗
...you did things that were unusual for you or that other people might have thought were excessive, foolish, or risky?		✗
...spending money got you or your family in trouble?	✗	
If you checked YES to more than one of the above, have you experienced several of these during the same period of time?		
How much of a problem did any of these situations cause you (like being unable to work; having family, money, or legal problems; and or getting into serious arguments/fights)? ☐ No problem ☐ Minor problem ☒ Moderate problem ☐ Serious problem		
Please discuss the results of this questionnaire with your physician.		

Clinician: *"Holly endorsed 6 of 13 manic symptoms, which constitutes a negative screen. In primary care, MDQ sensitivity was roughly 60 percent; thus false negatives may well occur. From here, I would go back and further question her on the items she did endorse by asking, 'Tell me about the time when you were hyper, what were you thinking about?' I would ask her husband, 'What is it like when she's this way?'" For example, during the periods of energy she might describe heading to the craft store to spend money on some project that she abandons as not being a good idea the next day. The interest and motivation never last long enough to get a project done."*

"In this way, the MDQ responses become a template for more targeted questioning and increasing enhancement of clinical interviewing skills for this complex illness."

References for Chapter 6

1. McElroy SL, Frye MA, Suppes T, et al. Correlates of overweight and obesity in 644 patients with bipolar disorder. *J Clin Psychiatry*. 2002;63:207–13.

2. Talbot F, Nouwen A. A review of the relationship between depression and diabetes in adults: is there a link? *Diabetes Care*. 2000;23:1556–62.

3. Cassidy F, Ahearn E, Carroll BJ. Elevated frequency of diabetes mellitus in hospitalized manic-depressive patients. *Am J Psychiatry*. 1999;156:1417–20.

4. American Psychiatric Association, American Psychiatric Association Task Force on DSM-IV. *Diagnostic and Statistical Manual of Mental Disorders: DSM-IV-TR*. Washington, DC: American Psychiatric Association; 2000.

5. Simon GE, VonKorff M, Piccinelli M, et al. An international study of the relation between somatic symptoms and depression. *N Engl J Med*. 1999 Oct 28;341(18):1329–35.

6. Frye MA, Calabrese JR, Reed ML, et al. Use of health care services among persons who screen positive for bipolar disorder. *Psychiatr Serv*. 2005 Dec;56(12):1529–33.

7. Ghaemi SN. Bipolar disorder and antidepressants: an ongoing controversy. *Primary Psychiatry,* 2001;8:28–34.

8. Bauer MS, Whybrow PC, Gyulai L, et al. Testing definitions of dysphoric mania and hypomania: prevalence, clinical characteristics and inter-episode stability. *J Affect Disord*. 1994;32(3):201–11.

9. Lish JD, Dime-Meenan S, Whybrow TC, et al. The National Depressive and Manic-depressive Association (DMDA) survey of bipolar members. *J Affective Disord*. 1994;31:281–94.

10. Hirschfeld RM, Lewis L, Vornik LA. Perceptions and impact of bipolar disorder: how far have we really come? Results of the National Depressive and Manic-depressive Association 2000 survey of individuals with bipolar disorder. *J Clin Psychiatry*. 2003;64:161–74.

11. Montano CB. Recognition and treatment of depression in a primary care setting. *J Clin Psychiatry*. 1994;55(Suppl):18–34.

12. Katzow JJ, Hsu DJ, Ghaemi SN. The bipolar spectrum: a clinical perspective. *Bipolar Disord*. 2003;5:436–42.

13. Akiskal HS, Bourgeois ML, Angst J, et al. Re-evaluating the prevalence of and diagnostic composition within the broad clinical spectrum of bipolar disorders. *J Aff Disord*. 2000;59:S5–30.

14. American Psychiatric Association. Practice guideline for the treatment of patients with bipolar disorder (revision). *Am J Psychiatry*. 2002;159(Suppl 4):1–50.

15. Frye MA, Gitlin MJ, Altshuler LL. Unmet needs in bipolar depression. *Depr Anx*. 2004;19:199–208.

INTRODUCTION

PRESENTATION

CLINICAL PROCESS

PHARMACOTHERAPY

RESOURCES

16. Slama F, Bellivier F, Henry C, et al. Bipolar patients with suicidal behavior: toward the identification of a clinical subgroup. *J Clin Psychiatry*. 2004 Aug;65(8):1035–9.

17. Michaelis BH, Goldberg JF, Davis GP, et al. Dimensions of impulsivity and aggression associated with suicide attempts among bipolar patients: a preliminary study. *Suicide Life Threat Behav*. 2004 Summer;34(2):172–6.

18. Raja M, Azzoni A. Suicide attempts: differences between unipolar and bipolar patients and among groups with different lethality risk. *J Affect Disord*. 2004;82(3):437–42.

19. Stuart MR, Lieberman JA 3rd. *The Fifteen-Minute Hour: Applied Psychotherapy for the Primary Care Physician*, 2nd ed. Westport, Conn.: Praeger Publications; 1993.

20. Lieberman JA 3rd, Stuart MR. The BATHE method: incorporating counseling and psychotherapy into the everyday management of patients. *Prim Care Companion J Clin Psychiatry*. 1999 Apr;1(2):35–8.

21. Akiskal HS, Benazzi F. Optimizing the detection of bipolar II disorder in outpatient private practice: toward a systematization of clinical diagnostic wisdom. *J Clin Psychiatry*. 2005 Jul;66(7):914–21.

22. McIntyre RS, Konarski JZ, Wilkins K, et al. The prevalence and impact of migraine headache in bipolar disorder: results from the Canadian Community Health Survey. *Headache*. 2006 Jun;46(6):973–82.

Chapter 7: Perform Differential Diagnosis/Evaluate Comorbidity

The range of mood presentations in bipolar illness and the highly individual course of the disorder often make accurate diagnosis a challenge. Comorbid disorders as well as those medical and psychiatric conditions with similar symptoms further complicate diagnosis.

This chapter addresses:

1. How bipolar disorder and conditions that present similar symptoms can be differentiated
2. What disorders tend to be comorbid with bipolar disorder
3. Treatment considerations for bipolar disorder and comorbid conditions

Conditions Relevant to Differential Diagnosis

When dysfunction is recognized, a thorough review of symptoms and medical history will assist in placing the dysfunction in a proper context, allowing other conditions to be considered in differential diagnosis and treatment planning. A variety of general medical and psychiatric conditions can present similar symptoms to bipolar disorder.

General Medical and Neurological Conditions

General medical and neurological conditions can produce alterations in mood that must be differentiated from manifestations of bipolar disorder. Some physiological causes to rule out are:

- **Embolic Stroke**, which occurs typically in an elderly individual. For example, parietal lobe strokes have been implicated in development of both depression and mania for some individuals.
- **Thyroid conditions**, which include hyperthyroidism (an excess of thyroid hormone), which can cause

In secondary mood disorders, the mood disturbance is determined to be the direct neurobiological consequence of a specific, often chronic, general medical/neurological disorder.

manic-like symptoms, or hypothyroidism (decreased thyroid hormone), which cause depression-like symptoms. Blood tests will indicate changes in hormone levels. Both conditions are associated with physical symptoms not usually observed in patients with bipolar disorder (e.g., elevated heart rate and blood pressure in hyperthyroidism and sensitivity to temperature change and skin bruises/tears in hypothyroidism).

- **Temporal lobe epilepsy**, which is associated with many of the same symptoms that can be seen in bipolar disorder — no coincidence since one of the main brain structures implicated in bipolar disorder is the brain's temporal lobe.

- **Neoplastic or cancer syndromes**, which can also be associated with some patients' change in usual presentation and development of bipolar-like symptoms.

See figure 7.1, below and on the next page, for medical conditions that can present as mood symptoms.

Figure 7.1   General Medical/Neurological Disorders that Can Present with Mood Symptoms

▲ **Metabolic Conditions**
- ◆ Vitamin B12 deficiency
- ◆ Porphyria
- ◆ Post-operative state
- ◆ Electrolyte abnormalities

▲ **Endocrinopathies**
- ◆ Hyperthyroidism/hypothyroidism
- ◆ Hyperparathyroidism/hypoparathyroidism
- ◆ Adrenocortical dysfunction
  (Addison's disease, Cushing's disease)

Figure 7.1   (continued)

▲ Infections
- ◆ Encephalitis
- ◆ Human immunodeficiency virus
- ◆ Hepatitis (A, B)
- ◆ Epstein Barr (infectious mononucleosis)
- ◆ Neurosyphilis
- ◆ Influenza
- ◆ Lyme disease

▲ Coronary Heart Disease

▲ Autoimmune/Connective Tissue Disorders
- ◆ Systemic lupus erythematosus
- ◆ Fibromyalgia

▲ Malignancy
- ◆ Carcinoma of the pancreas
- ◆ Multiple myeloma (calcium-related)

▲ Neurodegenerative Diseases
- ◆ Parkinson's disease
- ◆ Huntington's disease
- ◆ Alzheimer's disease

▲ Demyelinating Diseases
- ◆ Multiple sclerosis

▲ Other CNS Disease
- ◆ Stroke
- ◆ Right hemispheric lesions
- ◆ Closed-head injury
- ◆ Normal pressure hydrocephalus
- ◆ Cerebral sarcoidosis
- ◆ Tuberous sclerosis
- ◆ Familial cerebellar disease
- ◆ Idiopathic basal ganglia calcification
- ◆ Subcortical gray matter heterotopia

▲ Drugs
- ◆ Adrenal cortical steroids
- ◆ Isoniazid
- ◆ Disulfiram

INTRODUCTION

PRESENTATION

CLINICAL PROCESS

PHARMACOTHERAPY

RESOURCES

Depressive Disorders

Major Depressive Disorder with Irritable Mood

Many patients request help during depressive episodes, and if not queried specifically, clinicians may miss the history of hypomania or mania.

In some instances, the predominant mood in a patient with a major depressive disorder is not sadness, but rather irritability. Manifestations can include persistent anger, an exaggerated sense of irritation or frustration in response to minor annoyances, and a tendency to respond to events with angry outbursts or blaming others.[1] This presentation may be more common in children and adolescents.

It can be difficult to differentiate this presentation of depression from a manic episode with irritable mood, from mixed episodes, or from mixed or dysphoric hypomania, or even some forms of major depression.[2] The diagnosis requires a careful clinical evaluation to detect symptoms of hypomania or mania (e.g., decreased need for sleep, increased energy, impulsivity) and differentiate them from those of irritability with depression.

Patients with a major depressive episode may present seeking a sedative/ hypnotic as self-treatment for symptoms of mania, anxiety, and depression.

Clinicians in primary care should suspect bipolar disorder when irritability is the thematic or most troublesome symptom as well as a source of significant dysfunction at home or at work. Look for evidence of grandiose mood that imposes its desires or plans on other people or attempts to control and direct activities. The individual's past history and family history are important for developing a full picture of the symptoms.

Depressive symptoms need to be scrutinized for past, present, or future hypomanic, manic, or mixed symptoms to be differentiated from bipolar disorder.

Dysthymic Disorder

Dysthymic disorder is commonly found in a primary care setting and can present in children, adolescents, and adults. It is characterized by depressed mood for most of the day, for more days than not, for at least two years.[1] Criteria may be met by either self-report or by history obtained from others. Patients must have at least two of the following neurovegetative symptoms:

- Poor appetite or overeating
- Insomnia or hypersomnia
- Low energy or fatigue
- Low self-esteem
- Poor concentration or difficulty making decisions
- Feelings of hopelessness

Depression symptoms may include irritability, pessimism, and low social involvement. Differentiation of dysthymic disorder from a major depressive episode in a patient with bipolar disorder requires a history of mania or hypomania in the latter. In the absence of a history of mania/hypomania, a diagnosis of bipolar disorder cannot be made.

Dysthymic disorder is not part of the bipolar spectrum. Some data suggest that, in the presence of a first-degree relative with bipolar disorder, an early-onset dysthymia could be a prelude to a more full expression of bipolarity later in the illness course.

Longitudinal follow-up and careful assessment of treatment response is important in determining the actual diagnosis. Follow-up and treatment assessment should focus on spontaneous or perhaps treatment-emergent hypomania/mania.[3, 4] Treatment for dysthymic disorder consists of standard antidepressant strategies plus psychotherapy.[5]

INTRODUCTION

PRESENTATION

CLINICAL PROCESS

PHARMACOTHERAPY

RESOURCES

Substance-Related Disorders

Of all disorders with symptoms similar to bipolar disorder, probably substance-related disorders are the most common. The basis for this association may be one or more of the following:

1. Patients at risk for substance abuse disorder may also be at risk for bipolar disorder.

2. Substance abuse disorder may be genetically linked to the risk for bipolar disorder.

3. Chronic substance abuse may induce the development of mood symptoms and episodes.

4. Bipolar disorder is associated with poor impulse control, which can lead to more substance use.

5. Patients may be self-medicating affective symptoms.

Substance is a term used to refer to drugs of abuse, medications, and toxins. Those substances that, especially when abused, can cause bipolar-like (manic and/or depressive) symptoms include alcohol, cocaine and other stimulants, marijuana, other sedatives/hypnotics, opioids, inhalants, and corticosteroids. Substance-related disorders include substance dependence and withdrawal disorders, substance abuse, and substance intoxication. (See Figure 7.2 Substance-Induced Mood Disorders, Intoxication/Withdrawal on the next page.)

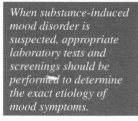

When substance-induced mood disorder is suspected, appropriate laboratory tests and screenings should be performed to determine the exact etiology of mood symptoms.

Figure 7.2   Substance-Induced Mood Disorders (Intoxication/Withdrawal)

Substance of Abuse	Bipolar-like Symptom Induced			
	Mood Swings	Irritability	Mania	Depression
Ethanol (Alcohol)	X	X		X
Cocaine/Other Stimulants	X	X	X	X
Marijuana	X	X		X
Other Sedatives/ Hypnotics		X		X
Opioids		X		X
Inhalants		X	X	X
Corticosteroids	X	X	X	X

Figure 7.3, below, summarizes typical clues for differentiating substance-related mood disorders from primary mood disorders.

Figure 7.3   Differential Clues to Substance-Related Mood Disorders

▲ **Suspect Substance-Related Mood Disorder if:**
   ◆ There is a history of substance abuse.
   ◆ Manifestations are typical of physiological/behavioral alterations associated with the substance.
   ◆ Onset and offset of clinical features are temporally related to substance use.
   ◆ Features and course are atypical for mood disorder.

▲ **Suspect Primary Mood Disorder if:**
   ◆ Mood symptoms persist more than two to four weeks after substance discontinuation.
   ◆ Dose of substance is unlikely to produce clinical manifestations.
   ◆ First degree relatives have a history of mood disorders.
   ◆ Prior mood episodes are unrelated to substance use.

INTRODUCTION

PRESENTATION

CLINICAL PROCESS

PHARMACOTHERAPY

RESOURCES

Alcohol Use

Alcohol, a CNS depressant, can potentiate the inhibitory actions of GABA and the receptor function of the excitatory amino acid NMDA. Because it also acts on a variety of other neurotransmitter systems, mood symptoms are common. Depression and insomnia that may suggest a major depressive disorder frequently accompany alcohol dependence and may even precede it.[1] Those with mild alcohol intoxication may have a sense of well-being and a bright expansive mood as ethanol levels rise. Following this period, depressive and/or anxiety symptoms may worsen over the next few hours or even the next day.

Stimulant Use

Stimulants producing altered mood states that mimic bipolar disorder manifestations include:

- Cocaine
- Amphetamines
- Methamphetamine
- Methylenedioxymethamphetamine (MDMA)

Figure 7.4, on page 103, presents the possible substance abuse symptoms/impacts and "street" names for many of these drugs.

Marijuana

Marijuana is made from dried portions of the cannabis plant. Its major psychoactive substance is tetrahydrocan-nabinol (THC). Consumption of THC by smoking or oral ingestion is associated with varying degrees of euphoria, laughter, and paramnesia. Initial wakefulness is followed by somnolence and lassitude. In moderate doses, marijuana may have anti-emetic effects and increase appetite. In higher doses, anxiety and psychosis can emerge, including paranoia, auditory, and visual hallucinations. Some users report enhanced levels of creativity.

Figure 7.4   Stimulants and Possible Symptoms

	Possible Symptoms	Impact
Cocaine and Amphetamines (crack, coke, speed, ice, meth)	• Intensive feelings of well being • Euphoria • Racing thoughts • Pressured speech • Hyperactivity • Increased sexual activity • Impulsive behavior • Grandiosity • Paranoia • Insomnia	• Inhibits dopamine reuptake into the nerve terminals via the dopamine transporter in the mesolimbic dopaminergic system and stimulates dopamine and other catecholamine release from pre-synaptic terminals[6] • May induce periods of depression/decreased energy after manic/hypomanic symptoms
MDMA (ecstasy, XTC, M&M)	• Euphoria • Empathy • Enhanced sociability • Increased energy • Memory loss • Depression • Impaired concentration • Poor sleep • Anxiety • Weight loss • Tremors • Paranoid psychosis (for typical recreational use over a long time) that is clinically indistinguishable from schizophrenia (reversible after patient is drug-free for an extended period)[9]	• May induce periods of depression/decreased energy after manic/hypomanic symptoms • May be toxic to sero-tonergic neurons, cells implicated in the pathophysiology of depression.[7] • May be taken by party-goers several times during an evening/night, which has been associated with structural abnormalities of the CNS[8]

Cannabis use is common in bipolar patients, but specific data on patterns of use, impacts, and adverse effects are lacking.[10] What research has been published suggests that:

- More men with bipolar disorder than women are users.[11]
- Marijuana abuse among bipolar patients has been associated with a higher degree of alcohol and other drugs of abuse.[12]
- Marijuana has been associated with the subsequent development of manic symptoms in the general population.[13]

Some have argued that the prevalence of marijuana use among bipolar patients suggests potential therapeutic effects for THC and cannabidiol and that randomized controlled trials may be warranted.[14]

In practice, patients with bipolar disorder may use marijuana to induce sleep or reduce irritable mood and to maintain emotional control. However, the patient may fail to connect the initial euphoria experienced to later effects — including exacerbation of anxiety or dysphoria.

Intoxication with Sedatives and Hypnotics

Sedatives, such as the benzodiazepines, that have a rapid onset (e.g., diazepam and alprazolam) tend to both be popular among drug abusers seeking the drugs' ability to produce a "high" and are the most commonly prescribed drugs in the world.[7] Barbiturates and non-benzodiazepine medications can also produce similar symptoms. Withdrawal symptoms mimic mania (e.g., anxiety, agitation, and delirium). Methaqualone ("Quaalude," "Lude"), classified as a schedule I substance since the early 1980s, is easily synthesized and sold for its psychoactive effects. Symptoms of intoxication and withdrawal are similar to those of other sedative/hypnotics. Figure 7.5, on the following page, covers sedative abuse.

Figure 7.5   Sedatives and Possible Symptoms

	Possible Symptoms	Impact
Gamma hydroxybutyrate (Easy Lay, Georgia Home Boy, and Liquid Ecstasy, "date rape" drug)	• Mood alterations (e.g., euphoria) • Hallucinations • Amnesia • Intensified effects of other drugs	• A CNS depressant • "Date rape" drug
Flunitrazepam (Rohypnol) (La Roche, Roofies, Mexican Valium, and "date rape" drug)	• Euphoria • Depersonalization • Emotional withdrawal/inebriation • Decreased pain perception • Manic-like and psychotic symptoms (dose dependent)	• No longer available in U.S., but smuggled in from other countries • Unlike other benzodiazepines, it is not detected by standard enzyme-multiplied immunoassay technique (EMIT) procedure. Ketamine and PCP analogs may also escape detection in assays designed to identify PCP.

Opioid Abuse

As drugs of abuse, opioid intoxication can produce euphoria, tranquility, and other mood changes believed to be the effects of the drugs on mesolimbic dopaminergic pathways and the nucleus accumbens.[15] Intoxication can also produce CNS and respiratory depression. Withdrawal may be accompanied by dysphoria and irritability.

Although heroin is the most common opiate abused, significantly more potent designer derivatives of fentanyl and meperidine are manufactured in illegal laboratories.[9] Designer opioid intoxication typically shows up in a patient admitting to use but with a negative urinary opioid screen and mood alterations.

Corticosteroid Use

Corticosteroids are widely used to treat a variety of inflammatory and immune-mediated disorders as well as some hematologic malignancies. Symptoms of hypomania, mania, depression, and psychosis are possible during medically indicated corticosteroid therapy and are dose related.[16]

Most patients treated with supraphysiologic doses of glucocorticosteroids will respond with an elevation of mood and a sense of well-being that is disproportionate to the state of their disease and sometimes mimicking a manic or hypomanic state.[7] Psychotic manifestations may also occur; for some patients, glucocorticoids induce depressive symptoms, particularly with long-term use.

Anxiety Disorders

Severe anxiety disorders may also be mistaken for bipolar disorder. For multiple anxiety disorders, the prominent clinical presentation is chronic and debilitating anxiety, versus fluctuating mood episodes on the bipolar spectrum. Persons with anxiety disorders present as chronically worried or fearful, and have corresponding reductions in their ability to function as a result of those fears. Consultation with an expert in diagnosing and treating these conditions may be appropriate for solving this diagnostic conundrum.

Differential diagnosis with anxiety disorders can be complex, particularly given the high rate at which these conditions co-occur.[17] An individual presenting with anxiety, panic attacks, or post traumatic stress disorder must be evaluated for bipolar disorder.[18] Similarly, it is important to differentiate general anxiety from hypomania as symptoms may sound similar (e.g., "racing thoughts," etc.). A key difference is the presence of increased energy with decreased sleep, unrelated to whether the mood state is euphoric, dysphoric, or irritable.

Other Psychiatric Disorders

Schizophrenia and Schizoaffective Disorder

Schizoaffective disorder consists of symptoms of schizophrenia and major affective disorder (e.g., bipolar disorder, major depressive disorder). The DMS-IV(TR) diagnosis of schizoaffective disorder requires an uninterrupted period of illness characterized by active symptoms of schizophrenia plus concurrent manifestations of either a major depressive disorder, manic episode, or mixed episode (manic, depressive).[1] During the course of schizoaffective symptoms, the patient must also experience delusions or hallucinations for at least two weeks **(in the absence of prominent mood symptoms)**. Lastly, mood symptoms should be present for a substantial portion of both the active and residual phases of the illness. Manic symptoms occur in the bipolar subtype of schizoaffective disorder, but the course of illness is distinguished by persistence of psychosis significantly beyond remission of mania.

> *The bipolar subtype of schizoaffective disorder differs from bipolar disorder in persistence of psychotic symptoms significantly beyond duration of mood episodes.*

Differentiation of mood disorder from schizophrenia can be difficult. Psychotic manifestations may be present in patients with bipolar disorder, and mood disturbances are common during all phases of schizophrenia. Depressive symptoms especially occur in patients with chronic psychotic disorders. To differentiate the two, it is important to carefully chart a longitudinal history of the symptoms. Psychotic manifestations of patients with bipolar disorder primarily manifest themselves during periods of mood instability while the total duration of mood symptoms is relatively brief in patients with schizophrenia. Since there are differences in therapy for the two disorders, it is important to establish a precise diagnosis.

If psychotic manifestations are present, do not assume that the patient has schizophrenia. It is important to remember that first-rank psychotic symptoms (hallucinations, thought

INTRODUCTION

PRESENTATION

CLINICAL PROCESS

PHARMACOTHERAPY

RESOURCES

broadcasting, etc.) can be seen in individuals experiencing mania. While psychotic manifestations may be present in patients with bipolar disorder, affective symptoms are not a major enduring component of schizophrenia. The diagnosis of schizophrenia should be one of exclusion of psychotic mood disorders.

Attention Deficit Hyperactivity Disorder (ADHD)

Attention deficit hyperactivity disorder (ADHD) is characterized by a persistent pattern of inattention and/or hyperactive-impulsivity that is more common and severe than that observed in other individuals at a comparable stage of development.[1] While typically considered a disorder predominantly of children, manifestations can persist into adulthood for about half of the individuals. Features of the disorder that may raise the possibility of bipolar illness include hyperactivity (as if "driven by a motor") and impulsivity. While these syndromic manifestations may be suggestive of mania, functional and social impairments of ADHD may contribute to depression.

Unlike other mood or psychotic disorders, ADHD can be diagnosed as a comorbid condition in those with bipolar disorder.

For individuals with ADHD, manifestations are often chronic and mixed. In bipolar disorder, manifestations are cyclic and euphoric or mixed, though it should be noted that, in children, bipolar disorder may present as more persistent and less cyclic. Family history of affective illness needs to be considered when evaluating a patient for ADHD versus bipolar disorder. Symptoms characteristic of mania (but not ADHD per se) include:

- Pressured speech
- Grandiosity or persistently elevated mood
- Decreased need for sleep
- Psychosis
- Racing thoughts

Early onset mania may represent a developmental subtype of bipolar disorder. Those children affected will typically meet criteria for ADHD during manic or mixed phases of illness.[19] Depressive episodes may complicate ADHD illness course. Patients with comorbid ADHD and bipolar depression appear to differ from those with unipolar depression in terms of more severe suicidality, anhedonia, hopelessness, and disruptive behavior disorders (e.g., conduct disorder, oppositional defiant disorder). The family histories of such patients also include greater psychiatric illness in first-degree relatives.[20]

Bipolar disorder and ADHD may be comorbid, and as such, may present a frequent clinical scenario.[21] Figure 7.6 on the next page presents some clues for differentiating between the two. More research is needed to characterize effective treatment of such patients. However, stabilization of bipolar disorder should ordinarily precede interventions aimed at ADHD.

Impulse Control Disorders

Impulse control disorders consist of a group of conditions that share the essential feature of being unable to resist an impulse, drive, or temptation to perform an action potentially harmful to the person or others.[1] In most instances, an individual with an impulse control disorder experiences an increasing sense of tension or arousal before committing the act. Impulse control disorders include kleptomania, pyromania, intermittent explosive disorder, and pathological gambling. Importantly, in patients with bipolar disorder, these activities are a component of mania or possibly hypomania.

Psychotic Disorder NOS

This is a residual diagnostic category for patients displaying brief (one day to one month) psychotic symptoms not better accounted for by another illness.

INTRODUCTION

PRESENTATION

CLINICAL PROCESS

PHARMACOTHERAPY

RESOURCES

**Figure 7.6   Differential Diagnosis of
Bipolar Disorder and ADHD**

Symptom or Feature	Bipolar Disorder	ADHD
Grandiosity	Present in manic phase	Absent
Decreased need for sleep	Present in manic phase	Absent
Abnormal Persistent Irritable Mood	Characteristic of mania	Not typical
Course of Illness	Episodic, but can be chronic persistent in children	Chronic persistent
Onset of Illness	Typically late childhood or adolescence	Less than age 7 by definition
Presistence into adulthood	Nearly always	In about 30–40%
Presence of psychosis	Possible	Absent

Differential Diagnostic Tools

To improve identification of patients with bipolar disorders, Hirschfeld et al. developed a three-part Mood Disorder Questionnaire (MDQ).[22] Subsequently, in collaboration with Dr. Hirschfeld, Compact Clinicals has developed the MDQ-Expanded, with additional features.[23] Other screening tools used frequently include the PHQ-9 (Patient Health Questionnaire) and the TEMPS-A (Temperament Evaluation of the Memphis, Pisa, Paris, and San Diego Autoquestionnaire).

Mood Disorders Questionnaire (MDQ)

The MDQ screens for a history of symptoms of mania or hypomania and the degree of functional impairment produced by these symptoms (No problem; Minor problem; Moderate problem; Serious problem).

Researchers initially validated the MDQ as a screening tool based on responses gathered from five psychiatric outpatient clinics primarily treating patients with mood disorders. In this study, a research professional, unaware of the MDQ results, conducted a telephone research diagnostic interview by using the bipolar module of the Structured Clinical Interview for DSM-IV. The MDQ demonstrated 73 percent sensitivity and 90 percent specificity for bipolar illness, when ≥7 symptoms were endorsed as occurring simultaneously and impairment was rated as either a "moderate" or "serious" problem.[22]

> *For primary care physicians, the MDQ can serve an important educational function. Using it helps one become more familiar with components of mania, which enhances clinical interviewing skills. This, in turn, may improve diagnostic accuracy and help patients develop greater insight into their illness.*

The MDQ has been subsequently validated by other investigators.[24] The sensitivity of the MDQ significantly decreases when used to screen the general population instead of outpatients with mood disorders.

Both a positive and negative MDQ warrants a more in-depth clinical interview. In the latter case, the patient's insight may be poor or their symptom recognition of hypomania may be low due to lack of psychoeducation. While not a perfect screening tool, the MDQ may be of value in primary care as a template from which to ask patients about past and current manic symptoms. Routine use may also be instructive in familiarizing primary care clinicians with elements of diagnosis and the clinical interview.[25] Using the MDQ along with other screening instruments in the assessment of patients with depression and anxiety is recommended.

INTRODUCTION

PRESENTATION

CLINICAL PROCESS

PHARMACOTHERAPY

RESOURCES

MDQ-Expanded

A new version of the Mood Disorder Questionnaire (MDQ-Expanded) offers screening for:[23]

- Current symptoms of mania (instead of only past ones)
- Depression
- Alcohol abuse

Other Tools

Other screening instruments for bipolar disorder include the PHQ-9 and the TEMPS-A. The PHQ-9 (Patient Health Questionnaire) is a screener for major depression that can be used to assess the presence and severity of depressive symptoms in patients with bipolar disorder. For more information, see pages 281–283 in section E.

The TEMPS-A (Temperament Evaluation of the Memphis, Pisa, Paris, and San Diego Autoquestionnaire), shows promise in the identification of bipolarity.[26] Its emphasis on mood lability and cyclothymia may improve recognition of patients with bipolar II disorder, even children and adolescents.[27, 28] The TEMPS-A can be used for further inquiry into the presence of cyclothymic traits (e.g., mood lability, dilletantism, etc.) common in patients with bipolar II disorder. It can also identify the presence of chronic hypomanic traits (hyperthymic temperament) that, in at least one study, have been associated with increased risk of antidepressant-emergent mania.[29] These and other validated assessment tools are covered in chapter 15.

HOLLY

Holly completed the MDQ. In her case, the MDQ is falsely negative (only 6 of 13 manic symptoms endorsed in question 1), but reveals significant numbers of symptoms that appear concurrently and are moderately impairing.

Holly has a history of major depression and is currently in an episode of moderate severity based her PHQ-9 score. She also experiences recurrent episodes of abnormally elated or irritable mood consistent with hypomania. There is no evidence at this time that she has experienced a period of marked impairment, lasting the one week necessary for a diagnosis of mania. Holly meets the criteria for bipolar II disorder.

Holly uses alcohol infrequently now, but has used alcohol binges in the past to "unwind" or sleep. Holly quite openly admits that her "current drug of choice is food." When her depression is prominent, she binges on sweets or other carbohydrates. She has only purged after a period of binging once – that was in high school. She has a history of panic attacks, unsuccessfully treated with antidepressants. She uses her clonazepam if she feels an attack is imminent.

Comorbidities in Patients with Bipolar Disorder

Relative to the general population, patients with bipolar disorder have higher lifetime prevalence rates for many medical and psychiatric illnesses, including; cardiovascular disease, cancer, obesity, type 2 diabetes mellitus (T2DM), substance abuse, anxiety disorders, personality disorders, and eating disorders. The presence of comorbidities can complicate the diagnosis and treatment of bipolar disorder by:

- Impairing functional outcomes
- Contributing to cyclic acceleration and more severe episodes over time
- Complicating treatment due to drug interaction or impaired organ function
- Requiring aggressive treatment of comorbidities to improve long-term outcomes

Medical Comorbidity

The presence of a comorbid medical condition interacts with bipolar disorder because:

- Medical conditions can both exacerbate and be exacerbated by bipolar disorder.
- Treatments for medical conditions and for bipolar disorder can exacerbate one another.

For example, the increased risk for obesity and T2DM, which can be exacerbated by weight gain from some bipolar disorder treatments, suggests that monitoring body weight, calculating body mass index (BMI), and learning about sound diet, nutrition, and exercise are important components of treatment.[30] (See chapter 10.)

Mood symptoms may be associated with general medical conditions or treatments for such conditions. Further, treatments for some medical conditions can influence the course of an existing mood disorder or the diathesis for a mood disorder or vice versa. In some cases, the comorbidity of general medical and psychiatric conditions are unrelated, but important in holistic management and outcome. Of recent interest are the links between bipolar illness and T2DM as well as that of mood disorders in general and the prevalence and morbidity of cardiovascular illness.

Thyrotoxicosis can create manic-like states. Hypothyroidism is associated with depression. Stroke is often associated with affective aberrations (as is epilepsy), closed head trauma, multiple sclerosis, HIV infection, and other conditions affecting the central nervous system. T2DM, asthma, and connective tissue disorders have all been reported to be associated with increased risk of depression.

Centrally acting antihypertensive agents, beta blockers, corticosteroids, histamine 2 blockers, anti-Parkinsonian agents, first generation antihistamines, and pro-motility agents for gastrointestinal conditions (e.g., metaclopramide) may have adverse effects on mood. Cancer chemotherapy is associated with both cognitive and mood changes in some patients. There is an increased risk of depression following coronary artery bypass grafting.

Recently published literature reviews suggest that patients with bipolar disorder may be predisposed to cardiovascular risk factors (e.g., obesity, smoking, hypertension, dylipidemia, metabolic syndrome, and T2DM).[31, 32] The ADA recommends close monitoring of metabolic parameters prior to and after the initiation of pharmacological treatment (see pages 172 through 176 in chapter 10 for detailed monitoring recommendations).

JANICE

With history of a concurrent manic episode and major depression, Janice was diagnosed with bipolar I disorder, most recent episode mixed.

Janice agreed to a voluntary inpatient admission for treatment based on her high suicide risk.

No baseline labs were done to establish the absence of medical comorbidity or mood disorders secondary to a general medical condition. Her doctor realized that lab work would be drawn at the hospital, as a reference point for future lab work (metabolic parameters in case atypical antipsychotics are used for treatment, CBC to get a baseline platelet count since divalproex was being considered, etc.). The hospital would also perform a urine drug screen in all likelihood.

INTRODUCTION

PRESENTATION

CLINICAL PROCESS

Psychiatric Comorbidity

The most common psychiatric comorbidities are substance-related, anxiety, personality, and eating disorders. In a 2001–2002 data analysis of 43,093 participants in the National Epidemiologic Survey

In patients with bipolar disorder who have a co-occurring substance abuse disorder, the diagnoses would be bipolar disorder and the specific substance abuse disorder.

PHARMACOTHERAPY

on Alcohol and Related Conditions, Grant et al. found that bipolar I disorder was "highly and significantly" associated with substance use (but not alcohol), anxiety, and personality disorders.[17] Baldassano et al., looking at the first 500 STEP-BD patients, found in a retrospective analysis that women with bipolar disorder had significantly higher rates of comorbid thyroid disease, bulimia, and post traumatic stress disorder, compared to men.[33] Schaffer et al., analyzed relevant data from the 2002 Canadian Community Health Survey: Mental Health and Well-Being, and found that substance use and anxiety disorders were very significantly associated with bipolar disorder.[34] The largest effect, according to this study, was for the presence of anxiety disorders (OR 7.94; 95%CI, 6.35-9.92). The high incidence of anxiety and mood disorder

RESOURCES

comorbidity was also established in the European Study of the Epidemiology of Mental Disorders (ESEMeD), in data derived from 21,425 responders.[18]

For the primary care physician, the common association of these psychiatric disorders with bipolar disorder has a number of practical implications.[35]

The presence of one axis I disorder is strongly associated with the existence or risk for other disorders. Substance abuse is particularly common, and anxiety disorders are increasingly recognized as comorbid with bipolar disorder and associated with poorer functional outcome and suicidality.[36, 37] Many in primary care are sensitive to anxious presentations and may be prone, just as in presentations that are more depressive, to jump to antidepressant therapy as a primary treatment option for the anxiety disorder. Primary care physicians are, therefore, cautioned not to be distracted by comorbid anxiety in the differential diagnosis of bipolar disorder. Some interventions for bipolar illness may be effective in reducing comorbid anxious symptoms.

Clinicians should evaluate:

- Comorbidities — Lifetime rates for illness prevalence and comorbidity with bipolar disorder are:
  - Substance use/abuse, 44 to 61 percent[35, 38]
  - Anxiety disorders, 24 to 42 percent[35, 39]
  - Personality disorders, 30 percent general prevalence (comorbidity is debated due to symptom overlap)
  - Eating disorders, 0.5 to 3 percent[35]
- Other psychiatric disorders that may be either diagnosed or emerge once a patient has been diagnosed with bipolar disorder, but not necessarily related to the bipolar disorder
- Children and adolescents for other Axis I disorder diagnostic criteria that may not have had sufficient time to evolve at first presentation of symptoms
- Patients presenting with substance-related, anxiety,

personality, impulse control, and eating disorders for symptoms diagnostic of a mood disorder

• Young people with a family history of mood disorders, including bipolar illness, with an early-onset anxiety, substance use, or eating disorder for a prodromal mood disorder including bipolar disorder

Psychosocial Context and Comorbidity

A clear view of psychosocial context is invaluable in understanding and planning interventions, especially when treating comorbid illness. Because bipolar illness is both severe and highly penetrant in families, patients often have the double burden of debilitating and labile extremes in mood, plus poor psychosocial support systems. Patients with bipolar disorder are "stormy," both internally and externally, often with chaotic circumstances reinforcing tendencies toward mood dysregulation and leading to maladaptive and psychosocially damaging behaviors. This kind of cycle supports the value of balanced biopsycho-social interventions that combine concurrent administration of proven pharmacologic agents, with psychoeducation and various psychotherapies or rehabilitation strategies.

For more information on these psychosocial interventions, see pages 187–190 of chapter 10.

INTRODUCTION

PRESENTATION

CLINICAL PROCESS

PHARMACOTHERAPY

RESOURCES

References for Chapter 7

1. American Psychiatric Association, American Psychiatric Association Task Force on DSM-IV. *Diagnostic and Statistical Manual of Mental Disorders: DSM-IV-TR*. Washington, DC; American Psychiatric Association: 2000.

2. Fava, M. Depression with anger attacks. *J Clin Psychiatry*. 1998;59(Suppl. 18):18–22.

3. Haykal RF, Akiskal HS. The long-term outcome of dysthymia in private practice: clinical features, temperament, and the art of management. *J Clin Psychiatry*. 1999 Aug;60(8):508–18.

4. Angst J, Gamma A, Benazzi F, et al. Toward a re-definition of subthreshold bipolarity: epidemiology and proposed criteria for bipolar-II, minor bipolar disorders and hypomania. *J Affect Disord*. 2003 Jan;73(1-2):133–46.

5. Bauer M, Whybrow PC, Angst J, et al. World Federation of Societies of Biological Psychiatry (WFSBP) Guidelines for Biological Treatment of Unipolar Depressive Disorders, Part 2: maintenance treatment of major depressive disorder and treatment of chronic depressive disorders and subthreshold depressions. *World J Biol Psychiatry*. 2002 Apr;3(2):69–86.

6. Tomkins DM, Sellers EM. Addiction and the brain: the role of neurotransmitters in the cause and treatment of drug dependence. *CMAJ* 2001;164(6):817–21.

7. Goodman LS, Hardman JG, Limbird LE, et al. *Goodman & Gilman's The Pharmacological Basis of Therapeutics*. New York; McGraw-Hill: 2001.

8. Buchanan JF, Brown CR. 'Designer drugs'. A problem in clinical toxicology. *Med Toxicol Adverse Drug Exp*. 1988;3(1):1–17.

9. Hibbs J, Perper J, Winek CL. An outbreak of designer drug-related deaths in Pennsylvania. *JAMA*. 1991;265(8):1011–3.

10. Brown ES, Suppes T, Adinoff B, et al. Drug abuse and bipolar disorder: comorbidity or misdiagnosis? *J Affect Disord*. 2001 Jul;65(2):105–15.

11. Kawa I, Carter JD, Joyce PR, et al. Gender differences in bipolar disorder: age of onset, course, comorbidity, and symptom presentation. *Bipolar Disord*. 2005 Apr;7(2):119–25.

12. Salloum IM, Cornelius JR, Douaihv A, et al. Patient characteristics and treatment implications of marijuana abuse among bipolar alcoholics: results from a double blind, placebo-controlled study. *Addict Behav*. 2005 Oct;30(9):1702–8.

13. Henquet C, Krabbendam L, de Graaf R, et al. Cannabis use and expression on mania in the general population. *J Affect Disord*. 2006 Oct; 95(1-3):103–10. Epub 2006 Jun 21.

14. Ashton CH, Moore PB, Gallagher P, et al. Cannabinoids in bipolar affective disorder: a review and discussion of their therapeutic potential. *J Psychopharmacol*. 2005 May;19(3):293–300.

15. Zocchi A, Girlanda E, Varnier G, et al. Dopamine responsiveness to drugs of abuse: A shell-core investigation in the nucleus accumbens of the mouse. *Synapse*. 2003;50(4):293–302.

16. Brown ES, Suppes T. Mood symptoms during corticosteroid therapy: a review. *Harvard Review of Psychiatry*. 1998;5(5):239–46.

17. Grant BF, Stinson FS, Hasin DS, et al. Prevalence, correlates, and comorbidity of bipolar I disorder and axis I and II disorders: results from the National Epidemiologic Survey on Alcohol and Related Substances. *J Clin Psychiatry*. 2005;66:1205–15.

18. Alonso J, Angermeyer MC, Bernert S, et al. 12-month comorbidity patterns and associated factors in Europe: results from the European Study of the Epidemiology of Mental Disorders (ESEMeD) project. *Acta Psychiatr Scand*. 2004:109(Suppl. 420):28–37.

19. Biederman J, Faraone SV, Wozniak J, et al. Clinical correlates of bipolar disorder in a large, referred sample of children and adolescents. *J Psychiatr Res*. 2005 Nov;39(6):611–22.

20. Wozniak J, Spencer T, Biederman J, et al. The clinical characteristics of unipolar vs. bipolar major depression in ADHD youth. *J Affect Disord*. 2004 Oct;82 (Suppl 1):S59–69.

21. Nierenberg AA, Miyahara S, Spencer T, et al. Clinical and diagnostic implications of lifetime attention-deficit/hyperactivity disorder comorbidity in adults with bipolar disorder: data from the first 1,000 STEP-BD participants. *Biol Psychiatry*. 2005 Jun;57(11):1467–73.

22. Hirschfeld RM, Williams JB, Spitzer RL, et al. Development and validation of a screening instrument for bipolar spectrum disorder: the Mood Disorder Questionnaire. *Am J Psychiatry*. 2000;157(11):1873–5.

23. Hirschfeld R. and Compact Clinicals. *Mood Disorder Questionnaire–Expanded*. Kansas City, Missouri: Compact Clinicals. 2005.

24. Hirschfeld RM, Holzer C, Calabrese JR, et al. Validity of the Mood Disorder Questionnaire: a general population study. *Am J Psychiatry*. 2003;160(1):178–80.

25. Manning JS. The Mood Disorder Questionnaire in primary care: (Not) ready for prime time? *Prim Care Companion J Clin Psychiatry*. 2002 Feb;4(1):7–8.

26. Akiskal HS, Akiskal KK, Haykal RF, et al. TEMPS-A: progress towards validation of a self-rated clinical version of the Temperament Evaluation of the Memphis, Pisa, Paris, and San Diego Autoquestionnaire. *J Affect Disord*. 2005 Mar;85(1-2):3–16.

27. Mendlowicz MV, Akiskal HS, Kelsoe JR, et al. Temperament in the clinical differentiation of depressed bipolar and unipolar major depressive patients. *J Affect Disord*. 2005 Feb;84(2-3):219–23.

28. Kochman FJ, Hantouche EG, Ferrari P, et al. Cyclothymic temperament as a prospective predictor of bipolarity and suicidality in children

INTRODUCTION

PRESENTATION

CLINICAL PROCESS

PHARMACOTHERAPY

RESOURCES

and adolescents with major depressive disorder. *J Affect Disord*. 2005 Mar;85(1-2):181–9.

29. Henry C, Sorbora F, Lacoste J, et al. Antidepressant-induced mania in bipolar patients: identification of risk factors. *J Clin Psychiatry*. 2001 Apr;62(4):249–55.

30. Citrome L, Jaffe A, Levine J, et al. Relationship between antipsychotic medication treatment and new cases of diabetes among psychiatric inpatients. *Psychiatr. Serv*. 2004 Sep;55(9):1006–13.

31. Newcomer JW. Medical risk in patients with bipolar disorder and schizophrenia. *J Clin Psychiatry*. 2006;67 (Suppl 9):25–30.

32. Taylor V, MacQueen G. Associations between bipolar disorder and metabolic syndrome: a review. *J Clin Psychiatry*. 2006 Jul;67(7):1034–41.

33. Baldassano CF, Marangell LB, Gyulai L, et al. Gender differences in bipolar disorder: retrospective data from the first 500 STEP-BD participants. *Bipolar Disorders*. 2005:7:465–70.

34. Schaffer A, Cairney J, Cheung A, et al. Community survey of bipolar disorder in Canada: lifetime prevalence and illness characteristics. *Can J Psychiatry*. 2006;51:9–16.

35. McElroy SL, Altshuler LL, Suppes T, et al. Axis I psychiatric comorbidity and its relationship to historical illness variables in 288 patients with bipolar disorder. *Am J Psychiatry*. 2001;158(3):420–6.

36. Otto MW, Simon NM, Wisniewski SR, et al. Prospective 12-month course of bipolar disorder in out-patients with and without comorbid anxiety disorders. *Br J Psychiatry*. 2006 Jul;189:20–5.

37. Simon NM, Otto MW, Wisniewski SR, et al. Anxiety disorder comorbidity in bipolar disorder patients: data from the first 500 participants in the Systematic Treatment Enhancement Program for Bipolar Disorder (STEP-BD). *Am J Psychiatry*. 2004 Dec;161(12):2222–9.

38. Regier DA, Farmer ME, Rae DS, et al. Comorbidity of mental disorders with alcohol and other drug abuse. Results from the Epidemiologic Catchment Area (ECA) Study. *JAMA*. 1990;264(19):2511–8.

39. Henry C, Van den Bulke D, Bellivier F, et al. Anxiety disorders in 318 bipolar patients: prevalence and impact on illness severity and response to mood stabilizer. *J Clin Psychiatry*. 2003;64(3):331–5.

Chapter 8:
Formulate a Working Diagnosis

Two main types of mood disorders — major depressive (unipolar) and manic depressive (bipolar) — have distinctive genetic and clinical characteristics. This chapter will focus on helping the clinician determine which form of what symptom subgroup exists among patients presenting in the clinical setting.

Validation for medical diagnoses relies on evaluating five factors: phenomenology (symptoms), pedigree (family history), longitudinal course, treatment response, and biologic markers. A summary of differential features of bipolar and unipolar depression using these factors appears in figure 8.1, on the next page. Key concepts related to bipolar diagnosis include:

- **Identification of symptoms associated with manic/hypomanic episodes and mixed states** — Symptoms can range from psychosis without other manic symptoms to prominent euphoria, grandiosity, or expansiveness typical of mania. In-between presentations can include hypomanic symptoms after taking an antidepressant, below-DSM threshold manic symptoms, dysphoria, or irritability.

- **Psychiatric comorbidity is the rule, not the exception** — This is especially true for substance abuse disorders, anxiety disorders, and personality disorders.

- **Diagnosing or excluding bipolar disorder is the primary task in the evaluation of every depressed or anxious patient** — Key factors for this decision process involve age of onset, illness course, response to medications, family history, and **any** evidence of manic/hypomanic episodes in the past.

Uncertainties are inevitable and diagnoses often carry a "working" status with revisions made as ongoing patient contact allows repeated inquiry for specific symptoms, corroborating (or elucidating) history from others, observation of treatment response, and longitudinal tracking of changes in the illness. Biologic markers that are sensitive and specific are not (yet) available for either bipolar disorder or major depression.

Figure 8.1   Comparison of Bipolar Disorders and Major Depression Diagnostic Factors

Validating Factor for Diagnosis	Bipolar Disorder	"Unipolar" Major Depression
Phenomenology (symptoms)	Manic, hypomanic, and mixed states occurring in an illness that is predominately depressive	Depression only
Pedigree (family history)	Strongly positive for impairing mood disorders	May be less positive for impairing mood disorders
Longitudinal course	Onset in childhood or adolescence > 90% recurrence without medication	Age of onset across lifespan
Treatment response	Non-response, unstable response, or emergence of manic symptoms secondary to antidepressant treatment	Response to antidepressant monotherapy

The DSM-IV(TR) lists four bipolar disorders in its bipolar category:[1]

- Bipolar I [divided into six criteria sets to specify the type of the most recent episode (e.g., manic)]
- Bipolar II
- Cyclothymia
- Bipolar disorder not otherwise specified (NOS)

Bipolar II, cyclothymia, and bipolar NOS are without separate episode-type criteria sets. However, a number of other criteria sets exist that can apply to all bipolar disorders and help to provide a comprehensive picture of the illness. For example, one of the bipolar disorder courses specified by DSM-IV(TR) is rapid cycling: a distinctive pattern that, despite its specific therapeutic and prognostic features, is **not** currently categorized as a specific subtype of bipolar disorder. The material that follows presents each of the bipolar diagnoses as well as DSM specifier information.

Bipolar I Disorder

The diagnosis of bipolar I disorder requires the presence of at least one manic episode, with or without a history of a prior major depressive episode.[1] Figures 8.2a through 8.2e (below and on the following pages) delineate the criteria for various diagnoses related to bipolar I disorder.

Figure 8.2a   Diagnostic Criteria for Bipolar I Disorder, Single Manic Episode

A. Presence of only one manic episode and no past major depressive episodes. If this is the first manic presentation and there is a history of major depressive episode(s) in past, then the diagnosis is bipolar disorder, most recent episode manic.

B. The manic episode is not better accounted for by schizoaffective disorder and is not superimposed on Schizophrenia, Schizophreniform Disorder, Delusional Disorder, or Psychotic Disorder Not Otherwise Specified.

Figure 8.2b Diagnostic Criteria for Bipolar I Disorder, Most Recent Episode Hypomanic

A. Currently (or most recently) in a Hypomanic Episode.

B. There has previously been at least one Manic Episode or Mixed Episode.

C. The mood symptoms cause clinically significant distress or impairment in social, occupational, or other important areas of functioning.

D. The mood episodes in Criteria A and B are not better accounted for by Schizoaffective Disorder and are not superimposed on Schizophrenia, Schizophreniform Disorder, Delusional Disorder, or Psychotic Disorder Not Otherwise Specified.

Figure 8.2c Diagnostic Criteria for Bipolar I Disorder, Most Recent Episode Manic

A. Currently (or most recently) in a Manic Episode.

B. There has previously been at least one Major Depressive Episode, Manic Episode, or Mixed Episode.

C. The mood episodes in Criteria A and B are not better accounted for by Schizoaffective Disorder and are not superimposed on Schizophrenia, Schizophreniform Disorder, Delusional Disorder, or Psychotic Disorder Not Otherwise Specified.

Figure 8.2d   Diagnostic Criteria for Bipolar I Disorder, Most Recent Episode Mixed

A. Currently (or most recently) in a Mixed Episode.

B. There has previously been at least one Major Depressive Episode, Manic Episode, or Mixed Episode.

C. The mood episodes in Criteria A and B are not better accounted for by Schizoaffective Disorder and are not superimposed on Schizophrenia, Schizophreniform Disorder, Delusional Disorder, or Psychotic Disorder Not Otherwise Specified.

Figure 8.2e   Diagnostic Criteria for Bipolar I Disorder, Most Recent Episode Depressed

A. Currently (or most recently) in a Major Depressive Episode.

B. There has previously been at least one Manic Episode, Mixed Episode.

C. The mood episodes in Criteria A and B are not better accounted for by Schizoaffective Disorder and are not superimposed on Schizophrenia, Schizophreniform Disorder, Delusional Disorder, or Psychotic Disorder Not Otherwise Specified.

Reprinted with permission of American Psychiatric Association, Diagnostic and Statistical Manual of Mental Disorders, Fourth Edition, Text Revision, Washington, D.C., American Psychiatric Association, 2000.

INTRODUCTION

PRESENTATION

CLINICAL PROCESS

PHARMACOTHERAPY

RESOURCES

BILL

The clinician compared Bill's presentation and history to the DSM-IV(TR) criteria for bipolar I disorder (most recent episode depressed). The results appear in figure 8.3 below.

Figure 8.3   Link between DSM Diagnostic Criteria and Bill's Presentation/History

DSM-IV(TR) Criteria – BD I (Most Recent Episode Depressed)	Bill's Presentation/History
Currently (or recently) in a major depressive episode	Bill described 3–4 years during which he had not felt his mood was ever normal. He experienced "unrelenting sadness" for several weeks at a time and extremely low motivation. "Right now, I don't care about anything. I feel 'dead' inside," he said. "I'd rather feel sad than be without any feelings at all."
At least 1 manic episode	Bill recalls intense and prolonged periods of great energy and activity that began during college. Bill had been diagnosed as having bipolar disorder in his late twenties, having been referred to a psychiatrist for evaluation of anger problems.
Symptoms not part of schizoaffective, delusional, or psychotic disorder	There is no evidence of schizoaffective, delusional, or psychotic disorder because Bill had no overt hallucinations, delusions, or other psychotic symptoms without co-occurring mood symptoms.

Bipolar II Disorder

A bipolar II disorder diagnosis requires the presence of at least one hypomanic episode, with a history of at least one prior major depressive episode.[1] (See figure 8.4 below.) There should be no history of a manic or mixed episode, since the presence of either signals a bipolar I diagnosis.

Figure 8.4 Diagnostic Criteria for Bipolar II Disorder

A. Presence (or history) of one or more major depressive episodes.

B. Presence (or history) of at least one hypomanic episode.

C. There has never been a manic episode or a mixed episode.

D. The mood symptoms in Criteria A and B are not better accounted for by schizoaffective disorder and are not superimposed on Schizophrenia, Schizophreniform Disorder, Delusional Disorder, or Psychotic Disorder Not Otherwise Specified.

E. The symptoms cause clinically significant distress or impairment in social, occupational, or other important areas of functioning.

Reprinted with permission of American Psychiatric Association, Diagnostic and Statistical Manual of Mental Disorders, Fourth Edition, Text Revision, Washington, D.C., American Psychiatric Association, 2000.

HOLLY

The clinician compared Holly's presentation and history to the DSM-IV(TR) criteria for bipolar II disorder. The results appear in figure 8.5 on the next page.

INTRODUCTION PRESENTATION CLINICAL PROCESS PHARMACOTHERAPY RESOURCES

Figure 8.5 Link between DSM Diagnostic Criteria and Holly's Presentation/History

DSM-IV (TR) Criteria – BD II	Holly's Presentation/History
≥ 1 depressive episodes	"I overdosed on pain pills when I was 13. I can remember being depressed even before that."
≥ 1 hypomanic episode	"I can sometimes go through periods — for a few days or a week or so — when I have a lot of energy and get lots of things done. I feel restless." "I need less sleep. Maybe only 3 hours. My mind moves so fast I can hardly keep up with thoughts. It makes it very hard to concentrate."
No manic episode or mixed state	Without presence or history of psychotic symptoms or evidence of need for hospitalization, it appears that Holly has not experienced a period of marked impairment needed for a diagnosis of mania.
Symptoms not part of schizoaffective, delusional, or psychotic disorder	There is no evidence of schizoaffective, delusional, or psychotic disorder because Holly had never experienced hallucinations, delusions, or other psychotic symptoms.
Symptoms cause clinically significant distress/impairment in important functional areas	"I'm occasionally happy during those times, but usually I'm angry. My family avoids me. My husband says it's like a storm that passes after a few days." Holly's husband indicates that the severity of the problem is a major detriment to their marriage.

Hypomania differs from mania in severity. By definition, it does not produce marked functional impairment or require hospitalization. For patients with bipolar II disorder, hypomanic symptoms during the episode do not mean that the patient will develop mania. Whereas for bipolar I, hypomania is an unstable state that may herald the development of mania.

Figure 8.6, on the following page, shows the associated features and clinical course of bipolar I vs. II disorder.

Because bipolar disorder is under-identified, symptoms of mania or hypomania should be investigated in any patient with apparent unipolar major depressive episode. Since manic and hypomanic symptoms may be pleasurable, patients may only seek medical advice at the time of a major depressive episode. Patients may be unable to remember manic or hypomanic episodes as such or may fail to differentiate them from normal mood states.

DSM-IV(TR) doesn't distinguish between euphoric and mixed or dysphoric hypomania (coded as hypomania, regardless of associated mood symptoms). However, many patients, when hypomanic, present with concurrent depressive symptoms ("dysphoric hypomania"), making differentiation from ongoing depressive symptoms difficult and often unidentified as hypomania. While many patients with bipolar II disorder may have a history of hypomanic episodes, what they may experience most often are transient hypomanic or dysphoric hypomanic symptoms. While hypomania is more common overall during the course of illness for bipolar I disorder, once hypomanic, the likelihood of mixed or dysphoric hypomania is the same for patients with either bipolar I or bipolar II disorder.[2]

Figure 8.6   Clinical Features of Bipolar I & II Disorders

Clinical Feature	Bipolar I	Bipolar II
Gender	F = M*	F>M*
Mania	Yes	No
Hypomania	Yes (as a transitional state); more common in BDII (see previous page)	
Major depressive disorder (MDD) required for diagnosis	No	Yes
Psychotic symptoms[1]	• Yes, can occur during either phase • Does not occur during hypomania[1] • In both depression and mania, and possibly more common during manic and mixed episodes	
Completed suicide[2]	Same	Same
Rapid cycling incidence[3]	Same	Same
Relationship of manic/hypomanic episodes to MDD episode[4]	Same	Same
Time between episodes	May decrease with age**	

Notes: [1]Psychotic symptoms during hypomania move episode to be defined (by DSM-IV-TR) as mania. [2]Completed Suicide = 10% to 15%. [3]Rapid Cycling = 10% to 20%. [4]Relationship of manic/hypomanic episodes to major depressive episodes — 60% to 70% immediately before or after.

* In males, the first episode is more likely to be manic; in females, the first episode is more likely to be depressive in nature. Generally, males experience more manic episodes throughout the lifetime of the disorder while females experience more depressive episodes.

** Between episodes, patients experience significantly reduced symptoms; however, many have residual, sub-syndromal symptoms that, if not treated, can contribute to functional impairment.

Cyclothymia

Cyclothymia is a chronic, fluctuating mood disorder with numerous hypomanic and mild depressive symptoms.[1] (See figure 8.7 on pages 131 through 132.) Both the hypomanic and depressive symptoms are of insufficient number, severity, pervasiveness, or duration to meet full criteria for a major depressive or hypomanic episode.

Figure 8.7   Diagnostic Criteria for Cyclothymic Disorder

A. For at least 2 years, the presence of numerous periods with hypomanic symptoms and numerous periods with depressive symptoms that do not meet criteria for a Major Depressive Episode. Note: In children and adolescents, the duration must be at least 1 year.

B. During the above 2-year period (1 year in children and adolescents), the person has not been without the symptoms in Criterion A for more than 2 months at a time.

C. No Major Depressive Episode, Manic Episode, or Mixed Episode has been present during the first 2 years of the disturbance. Note: After the initial 2 years (1 year in children and adolescents) of Cyclothymic Disorder, there may be superimposed Manic or Mixed Episodes (in which case both Bipolar I Disorder and Cyclothymic Disorder may be diagnosed) or Major Depressive Episodes (in which case both Bipolar II Disorder and Cyclothymic Disorder may be diagnosed).

D. The symptoms in Criteria A are not better accounted for by Schizoaffective Disorder and are not superimposed on Schizophrenia, Schizophreniform Disorder, Delusional Disorder, or Psychotic Disorder Not Otherwise Specified.

(continued)

INTRODUCTION

PRESENTATION

CLINICAL PROCESS

PHARMACOTHERAPY

RESOURCES

Figure 8.7   (continued)

E. The symptoms are not due to the direct physiological effects of a substance (e.g., a drug of abuse, a medication) or a general medical condition (e.g., hyperthyroidism).

F. The symptoms cause clinically significant distress or impairment in social, occupational, or other important areas of functioning.

Reprinted with permission of American Psychiatric Association, Diagnostic and Statistical Manual of Mental Disorders, Fourth Edition, Text Revision, Washington, D.C., American Psychiatric Association, 2000.

Cyclothymic disorder is usually chronic, and as many as 50 percent of patients will subsequently develop bipolar I or bipolar II disorder.[1] Importantly, the development of major depressive, hypomanic, or manic symptoms after two years of cyclothymic manifestations does not negate the diagnosis of cyclothymic disorder; instead, patients are diagnosed with cyclothymic disorder plus the other major mood disorder.

Bipolar NOS

The bipolar NOS category is a residual diagnostic category for disorders with bipolar features that do not meet criteria for bipolar I, bipolar II, or cyclothymic disorder. A patient might experience multiple hypomanic episodes without inter-current major depressive episodes, or hypomanic and depressive symptoms may be too infrequent to qualify the patient for a cyclothymic diagnosis. In some instances, the NOS qualifier will be used while the clinician attempts to determine if the disorder is truly primary or is secondary to substances of abuse or a medical condition.

Diagnostic Specifiers for Bipolar Disorder

Diagnostic specifiers increase diagnostic specificity, aid in treatment selection, and improve prognostic accuracy. In addition, they also can improve the homogeneity of subgroups in clinical trials of bipolar disorder treatments and, thus, data analysis.

Specifiers Related to Episode, Onset, and Course

Bipolar disorder specifiers for the episode, onset, and course of the disorder have been developed and are listed in the DSM-IV(TR).[1] (See figures 8.8a, 8.8b, and 8.8c on pages 134 through 135.)

Special Notes on Rapid Cycling

Rapid cycling is an important course specifier for patients (with an established diagnosis of bipolar I or II disorder), who experience four or more mood episodes within a 12-month period that are either discrete, (i.e., demarcated by a partial or full remission of at least two months' duration); or characterized by a switch to an episode of opposite polarity.

Any subtype with a manic or hypomanic component is not considered to have "cycled." Thus, the disorders remain in the same pole when a mixed episode immediately follows a manic one, despite depressive symptomatology in the mixed episode. Another example would be severe depression changing to mild depression; symptoms would still be occurring at the same pole, and thus would not be considered to have switched.

Although bipolar disorder is gender neutral, women may be more likely to have a rapid cycling course than men. Rapid cycling episodes appear to be unrelated to the reproductive cycle or stage.

A rapid cycling course can be intermittent or persistent and can occur at any time during illness course. It is more common in patients with a variety of medical disorders, including hypothyroidism, neurological conditions, and mental retardation.[1]

INTRODUCTION

PRESENTATION

CLINICAL PROCESS

PHARMACOTHERAPY

RESOURCES

Figure 8.8a Bipolar Disorder Specifiers for Episode

Specifier	Comments
Severity	• Mild, moderate, or severe
Psychotic	• With or without psychotic symptoms
Remission	• In partial or full remission
Chronic	• Applied to mood disorder with a major depressive episode (i.e., major depression; bipolar I, most recent episode depressed; or, bipolar II, depressed)
Catatonic	• Motoric immobility or excessive purposeless motor activity • Extreme negativism • Peculiarities of voluntary movement • Echolalia or echopraxia
Melancholic	• Near complete absence of the capacity for pleasure • Present at nadir • Distinctively different than sadness or non-melancholic depression
Atypical Depression	• Mood reactivity — mood brightens in response to positive events • Significant weight gain or increase in appetite • Hypersomnia • Heavy, leaden feelings in arms and/or legs • Long-standing; impairment resulting from sensitivity to rejection

Figure 8.8b Bipolar Disorder Specifiers for Onset

Specifier	Comments
Post-partum	• Onset of major mood disorder within 4 weeks post-partum

Figure 8.8c   Bipolar Disorder Specifiers for Course

Specifier	Comments
With or Without Inter-episode Recovery	• With full-recovery • Without full-recovery
Seasonal Pattern*	• With or without • Regular, temporal relationship between major mood disorder onset and season • Seasonal, full-remission • Two seasonal major depressive episodes in 2 years • Seasonal major depressive episodes significantly outnumber nonseasonal ones during one's lifetime
Rapid Cycling	• Applied to bipolar I or II disorder • ≥4 episodes of mood disturbance in previous 12 months that meet criteria for major mood episode • Episodes have partial or full remission for at least 2 months, or there is a switch to an episode of opposite polarity

* DSM-IV(TR) discusses a seasonal depressive pattern only, but it is well recognized that seasonal patterns exist for hypomania and mania for some patients.

Reprinted with permission of American Psychiatric Association, Diagnostic and Statistical Manual of Mental Disorders, Fourth Edition, Text Revision, Washington, D.C., American Psychiatric Association, 2000.

INTRODUCTION

PRESENTATION

CLINICAL PROCESS

PHARMACOTHERAPY

RESOURCES

References for Chapter 8

1. American Psychiatric Association, American Psychiatric Association Task Force on DSM-IV. *Diagnostic and Statistical Manual of Mental Disorders: DSM-IV-TR*. Washington, DC: American Psychiatric Association; 2000.

2. Suppes T, Mintz, J, McElroy SL, et al. Mixed hypomania in 908 patients with bipolar disorder evaluated prospectively in the Stanley Bipolar Treatment Network: A gender-specific phenomenon. *Archives of General Psychiatry.* 2005 Oct;62:1089–96.

Chapter 9: Form Collaborative/ Therapeutic Treatment Alliances

Treating patients with bipolar disorder is challenging. Discontinuities and lack of integration in the delivery of health care further amplify those challenges. Many primary care clinicians are interested in providing excellent care to their patients with significant mental illness and fostering better communication and shared care with their colleagues in psychiatry and the specialty mental health setting. Effective collaborative care involves developing therapeutic treatment alliances with other health care professionals, with the patient, and often with significant others in the patient's life in order to develop a successful treatment plan.

Collaborative Care – A Primary Care Perspective

Once the existence of a bipolar disorder has been established, individual primary care physicians will typically determine a desired level of intervention based on various factors, such as practice setting, current and desired clinical skill set, and severity of illness. For these clinicians, there are three general categories of interventions:

1. **Patients who need immediate referral** — These will usually be patients with acute suicidal or homicidal ideation in need of inpatient or intense outpatient care. These patients need acute stabilization and monitoring while arrangements for further care are made.

   Other reasons for referral include illness that is beyond one's scope of practice and comfort level or problems with transference (displacement of feelings toward others onto the clinician) or counter transference (surfacing of a clinician's own feelings through identification with the emotions, experiences, or problems of the person undergoing treatment).

2. **Patients who can be transitioned to specialty care** — These patients will have illnesses judged to be beyond the primary care clinician's scope of practice or skill set for long-term care, but difficulties inherent in the referral process require the institution of evidence-based, short-term treatment.

3. **Patients who will not be referred to specialty care** — These patients will be judged candidates for ongoing care in a primary care settting. Consultation should be considered at critical decision points, such as when there exists:

   • *Some diagnostic dilemma* — Are presenting symptoms, history, assessment measure scores, and reports from significant others just not in sync?

   • *Treatment refractory status* — Are patients just not significantly better at follow up?

   • *The emergence of problematic transference or counter transference* — Do you just no longer feel good about the relationship for intangible reasons?

   • *A change in acuity/severity* — Could this patient's treatment needs be beyond my practice scope and available time?

   In such consultation situations, the primary care physician will need to take the lead in setting short- and long-term goals.

Obstacles to referral and consultation include:

1. **Scarcity** — In rural areas particularly, there may be limited numbers of psychiatrists or mental health centers.

2. **Long waiting times or great distance** — It may take weeks or months for less acutely ill patients to obtain appointments in the specialty sector. Distance and transportation problems may present significant obstacles.

3. **Financial barriers** — Lack of insurance parity may make specialty mental health care prohibitively expensive. Mental health carve-outs may limit "in-network" providers and other options.

4. **Negative stigma originating with the patient and provider** — Patients may resist referral to avoid negative labels about symptom origins. Mental health providers themselves may be viewed negatively, and primary care clinicians may overtly or covertly reinforce these stereotypes.

There may be times when absolutely no referral resources exist for care in the specialty mental health sector. In those situations, close attention to treatment guidelines and collaboration with informal sources of treatment support (e.g., pastoral care, 12-Step, etc.) may add helpful psychosocial support. Medical strategies that offer broad efficacy across diagnostic spectra (e.g., atypical antipsychotics for bipolar disorder, schizoaffective disorder, schizophrenia etc.) may be helpful. Clinicians now have access to continuing medical education online. In the future, telemedicine via video conferencing offers the potential to bridge gaps in consultation availability.

Shared care arrangements — where a primary care physician and psychiatrist more closely collaborate through a formal or informal network — offer advantages for everyone involved, including:

1. Patients benefit from an increased intensity of focus on a complex illness and from open communications between primary care and mental health providers.

2. Referring providers may learn through focused questions to experts how to improve and expand their own clinical skills and build professional relationships that benefit patients.

3. Mental health care practitioners benefit by the demystification of mental illness and providers.

INTRODUCTION

PRESENTATION

CLINICAL PROCESS

PHARMACOTHERAPY

RESOURCES

The reality is, of course, that psychiatric and general medical illness are usually comorbid and negatively impact each other and overall health. Psychiatric illness is often the doorway of declining health through comorbidity with diabetes mellitus, cardiovascular dysfunction, cancer, accidental death, and a neglect of lifestyles and health maintenance activities that may preserve or enhance overall health.

Models of Collaborative Care

Several models of collaborative care have been researched, though research on such interventions is limited at present. These interventions have included:[1-4]

- Co-location of PCP and mental heath care providers
- Provision for care managers dedicated to monitoring mental health, psychoeducation programs, brief psychotherapy, telephone follow-up, and practice arrangements that reduce barriers to consultation
- Focus on the acute treatment phase or treating patients with persistent symptoms

In major depression, such interventions have yielded greater symptom reduction, less impairment, and better quality of life in acute-phase interventions as well as improved adherence, satisfaction with care, and better depressive outcomes in patients with persistent depressive symptoms beyond the acute phase.[1, 2] In one study, acute-phase effects failed to persist in the following year.[5] A trial in patients with depression and diabetes improved depression outcomes, but not glycemic control.[3] Integrated primary care within a VA psychiatric clinic yielded improvements in the 36-item Short-Form Health Survey (SF-36) and a greater likelihood of receiving preventative measures outlined in clinical care guidelines, but patients did not improve in psychiatric symptom measures.[6]

Increasingly, integrated models of training and practice are advocated.[7, 8] Medical cost offsets may be achievable while providing improvements in outcome.[8]

Primary care providers can contribute to a collaborative relationship with mental health specialists by:

1. Ensuring that routine health maintenance and risk factor assessment don't get "lost" in the mental illness. Pap smears, immunizations, mammograms, and colorectal cancer screening can be emphasized. Risk assessment, screening, and interventions for coronary artery disease and diabetes mellitus can be made. Smoking cessation can be encouraged and supported.

2. Encouraging shared patients to "invest" their improvement in mental health in behaviors that enhance overall health (e.g., regular exercise, weight control, or participation in community activities).

   Additionally, the clinician can probe whether or not patients are willing to "invest" in making other changes related to their illness. Are they willing to get treatment for comorbid substance abuse? Would they be willing to try workplace strategies to lessen stress in their lives, or perhaps change jobs to avoid frequent travel or shift work?

3. Monitoring the status of psychiatric illness and encouraging early recognition of escalating severity of illness or danger to self/others. It should be noted that many patients who attempt or complete suicide visit a primary care physician in the month(s) prior to the act.[9-10]

4. Monitoring treatment for efficacy, safety, and tolerability by assisting those in psychiatry to monitor the impact of treatment on medical comorbidity or risk status, and, when necessary, managing those comorbidities in a manner that is respectful of the mental illness.

INTRODUCTION

PRESENTATION

CLINICAL PROCESS

PHARMACOTHERAPY

RESOURCES

The Therapeutic Alliance with the Patient

Establishing a positive therapeutic alliance with the patient requires individualized treatment, taking people where they are in the longitudinal course of the illness and working with them to achieve agreement about the treatment direction. By working together and tracking response to the evidence-based recommendations, patients will more likely feel like they are active participants in the treatment process.

Patients who are not a danger to themselves or others and who have the capacity to make decisions regarding their care may accept or decline treatment. For many, awareness and acceptance of any illness requires time. Primary care clinicians may be uniquely positioned to assist patients in this acceptance process by:

- Providing education and support from an "ally" that facilitates the efforts of colleagues in the specialty mental health sector
- Making empathetic inquiries into a patient's fund of knowledge, concerns, and readiness
- Repeatedly discussing and documenting the potential risks, benefits, adverse effects, and rationale of treatment

Specific provider factors that may contribute to improving the therapeutic alliance include: active participation by the patient in establishing visit agendas, empathy, good eye contact, "open" posture, an active listening style with frequent repeating of key patient statements asking for clarification, and demonstrations of respect for the patient, including cultural sensitivities. The use of the BATHE method previously discussed is a good framework for fostering a therapeutic alliance in the primary care setting, where interactions may be time limited.

Not only a strategy for patient assessment, the BATHE process (see page 81 in chapter 6) can enhance the therapeutic alliance.

BILL

Bill requested a refill of his methylphenidate prescription. Unfamiliar and uncomfortable with the use of psychostimulants in mood disorder patients, Bill's primary care physician recommended a psychiatric consultation.

The consulting psychiatrist discussed several treatment options, including optimization of the olanzapine-fluoxetine combination (OFC) dose. If residual depression was a problem, the fluoxetine component could be increased (6/25 to 6/50) If maintenance doses of olanzapine were needed, the combination could be 12/25, or both components could be increased to 12/50.

The psychiatrist felt the residual concentration difficulties might be related to incomplete resolution of Bill's depression. Psychostimulants, such as methylphenidate, could be considered if attention deficit symptoms persisted in the absence of depression.

Bill elected to begin lithim in addition to OFC. His dose was titrated to 1200 mg daily over two weeks. A lithium level at that dose was 0.9 mEq/l. His depression completely ameliorated over three months. His attention problems were also attenuated. He found that once his motivation and sleep completely improved, his attention difficulty also improved and required no further intervention.

Alliances with Patient Support Systems

Involving significant others as early as the initial interview can be helpful for optimizing overall care of the patient with bipolar disorder. Encouraging the selection and active participation of an "illness partner" may increase the retention of therapeutic messages and foster earlier interventions in the case of symptomatic relapse. Inviting a spouse or other close friend to be present for the entire conversation, to read informational handouts and ask questions about them is important, not just to gain their verbal perspective, but also to watch for nonverbal clues about the level of impairment symptoms cause in the relationship and other functional areas.

INTRODUCTION

PRESENTATION

CLINICAL PROCESS

PHARMACOTHERAPY

RESOURCES

Additionally, observing the dynamic between family members can illuminate communication and relationship issues that would best be served with referral to marriage/couple counseling.

One particular intervention, family-focused therapy (FFT) can be very useful. FFT is a psychoeducational intervention in which patients and relatives learn about bipolar disorder, the biopsychosocial model of illness, and the importance of medication adherence. Stress reduction is emphasized through strategies to reduce negative expressed emotion. Active listening, instruction in constructive criticism, and promotion of family brainstorming sessions encourage an atmosphere of partnership and supportive care.

> *Involvement of others allows the clinician to make those persons allies that can help keep the patient on track during days of pessimism, despondency, and self-doubt, when they might want to give up treatment prematurely.*

FFT has been shown in randomized trials to reduce episode relapse and improve depressive symptomatology. It was also associated with improvements in medication compliance. A comparison of FFT with individual psychotherapy demonstrated FFT superiority in fewer relapses and hospitalizations during the second year of observation.[11, 12]

> *For the primary care physician, understanding the nature of patient support systems may indicate whether or not the patient will likely be more difficult to treat and have more potential for labile moods and unexpected shifts into dangerous territory.*

The Impact of Treatment Alliances on Adherence

The quality of the therapeutic alliance has been shown to have an important impact on treatment adherence. In the NIMH Depression Collaborative Research program, this effect was observable in patients receiving both interpersonal and cognitive psychotherapy and in patients treated with an antidepressant or placebo alone.[13]

One factor significant for the patient may be expectancy of treatment outcome. Clearly, treatment outcome must be closely associated with treatment adherence. Part of the difficulty surrounding adherence is the perception of the patient that, once symptoms improve, they might not need to continue medications. Thus, it is vital that providers carefully communicate hope and a commitment to be an advocate in what will be a lifelong treatment journey.[14]

HOLLY

When discussing treatment options with Holly (who has just been diagnosed with bipolar II disorder), the primary care physician used a series of questions and affirmations to establish a positive anticipation about treatment.

> **Clinician**: *"Holly, you don't just have downs, you have ups and downs, and we have to treat the downs in people who have theses ups and downs in a very, very different way to get them to be better."* This helps set the stage for why treatment for someone with BDII may be different than experienced in the past (when diagnosed with major depression).

> **Holly**: *"Do you think I'm bipolar?"*

> **Clinician**: *"Yes, but not classically. You know, your family history includes some pretty solid evidence that some people have had manfestations of classic manic depressive illness. When we research this, we find that children of people with classic manic depressive illness very often have to be treated in different ways because they share features of bipolar illness that make their treatment different."* This approach acknowledges the genetic component but helps soften any stigma about not wanting to be diagnosed the same as a mother, father, or other relative.

> **Clinician**: *"How do you feel about being treated? What would you be interested in?"* For Holly, a different approach to treatment — one that might be more long-lasting in its therapeutic effect — was very hopeful.

Clinician: *"Holly, we are going to approach your treatment in a totally different way. I know you've had bad experiences with treatment of your depression in the past, but my sense is that those bad results were based on an unfocused diagnosis. I think the treatment probably hasn't been quite as targeted as we might make it. Are you interested in treating this depression in a different way; hopefully, with a better outcome?"*

Holly: *"Can I just deal with you for treatment; I don't want to have to go see anyone new."*

Clinician: *"I feel very comfortable beginning treatment for you, but I must be honest that I'm not a psychiatrist. I understand this illness pretty well, but if you get sick and become a danger to yourself or others, or develop other symptoms of great concern, I'm going to want you to be treated in a different place by a different person. If I run out of reasonable things to do, I'm going to want to refer you to somebody who has more reasonable things to do than I have."* This approach sets the stage for referral and consultation in the future as part of a positive collaborative approach.

References for Chapter 9

1. Unutzer J, Katon W, Callaghan CM, et al. Collaborative care management of late-life depression in the primary care setting: a randomized controlled trial. *JAMA*. 2002 Dec;288(22):2836–45.

2. Katon W, Von Korff M, Lin E, et al. Stepped collaborative care for primary care patients with persistent symptoms of depression: a randomized trial. *Arch Gen Psychiatry*. 1999 Dec;56(12):1109–15.

3. Katon WJ, Von Korff M, Lin EH, et al.The Pathways Study: a randomized trial of collaborative care in patients with diabetes and depression. *Arch Gen Psychiatry*. 2004 Oct;61(10):1042–9.

4. Roy-Byrne PP, Craske MG, Stein MB, et al. A randomized effectiveness trial of cognitive-behavioral therapy and medication for primary care panic disorder. *Arch Gen Psychiatry*. 2005 Mar;62(3):290–8.

5. Lin EH, Simon GE, Katon WJ, et al. Can enhanced acute-phase treatment of depression improve long-term outcomes? A report of randomized trials in primary care. *Am J Psychiatry*. 1999;156(4):643–5.

6. Druss BG, Rohrbaugh RM, Levinson CM, et al. Integrated medical care for patients with serious psychiatric illness: a randomized trial. *Arch Gen Psychiatry*. 2001 Sep;58(9):861–8.

7. Manning JS, Zylstra RG, Connor PD. Teaching family physicians about mood disorders: a procedure suite for behavioral medicine. *Prim Care Companion J Clin Psychiatry*. 1999 Feb;1(1):18–23.

8. Kathol R, Stoudemire A. Chapter 38. Strategic integration of inpatient and outpatient medical-psychiatry services. In: JR WMR, ed. *The Textbook of Consultation-Liaison Psychiatry*. Chapter 38. Second ed. Washington, DC: APPI Press; 2002.

9. Luoma JB, Martin CE, Pearson JL. Contact with mental health and primary care providers before suicide: a review of the evidence. *Am J Psychiatry*. 2002;159:909–16.

10. Andersen UA, Andersen M, Rosholm JU, et al. Contacts to the health care system prior to suicide: a comprehensive analysis using registers for general and psychiatric hospital admissions, contacts to general practitioners and practicing specialists and drug prescriptions. *Acta Psychiatr Scand*. 2000;102:126–34.

11. Miklowitz DJ, George EL, Richards JA, et al. A randomized study of family-focused psychoeducation and pharmacotherapy in the outpatient management of bipolar disorder. *Arch Gen Psychiatry*. 2003;60:904–12.

12. Rea MM, Tompson MC, Miklowitz DJ, et al. Family focused treatment vs. individual treatment for bipolar disorder: results of a randomized clinical trial. *J Consult Clin Psychol*. 2003;71:482–92.

13. Krupnick JL, Sotsky SM, Simmens S, et al. The role of the therapeutic alliance in psychotherapy and pharmacotherapy outcome: findings in the National Institute of Mental Health Treatment of Depression Collaborative Research Program. *J Consult Clin Psychol*. 1996 Jun;64(3):532–9.

14. Meyer B, Pilkonis PA, Krupnick JL, et al. Treatment expectancies, patient alliance, and outcome: further analyses from the National Institute of Mental Health Treatment of Depression Collaborative Research Program. *J Consult Clin Psychol*. 2002 Aug;70(4):1051–5.

INTRODUCTION

PRESENTATION

CLINICAL PROCESS

PHARMACOTHERAPY

RESOURCES

Chapter 10:
Select Treatment Modalities

As a lifetime illness, bipolar disorder should be treated like any other recurrent condition, with the general treatment goals being those of producing symptomatic remission, restoring full psychosocial functioning, and preventing relapse.

Both pharmacological and non-pharmacological options exist for the treatment of bipolar illness. As in other multi-factorial chronic illnesses, such as diabetes mellitus and asthma, the optimal management of bipolar disorder requires the efforts of a multidisciplinary team. Psychiatrists, primary care clinicians, nurses, psychotherapists, clinical pharmacists, social workers, and others all have a valid role to play. For example, psychotherapists experienced in providing psychosocial education about bipolar illness play an important part in the overall treatment plan.

Treatment should be conducted as a therapeutic alliance between the patient and clinician, with both parties recognizing new episodes, instituting steps to optimize therapy, managing adverse events, and identifying mild (prodromal) changes in mood or behavior that may predict syndromal manifestations.

During the early phase of treatment, careful monitoring is important in order to maximize the benefits of pharmaco-therapy and prevent patients from harming themselves or others. This is particularly important in mania — a mood state that may limit patients' insight into how their behavior may bring harm to relationships, work, and financial stability. It should also be noted that the majority of attempted and completed suicides occur during depressive or mixed episodes.[1, 2]

One challenging aspect of treatment is that bipolar illness has, for many patients, an existential quality that makes differentiation of illness from a "normal" emotional state problematic. Defining "normal" for any individual may be difficult. The process takes time and requires ongoing supportive therapeutic alliances. Contributors to this existential quality can include early onset of mood dysregulation, chronicity of symptoms, the illness' roots in temperament, and the presence of supranormal states of mood. The last includes depressed states mingled with manic excitement, a state interpreted as angst accompanied by philosophical insight. Therefore, each individual's goal for treatment will be different, and the clinician must maintain a respect (within the limits of safety) for the patient's objectives in seeking treatment. As such, it is important to actively elicit the patient's agenda for treatment with questions, such as:

- "What concerns do you have about the effect of treatment on your personality? Relationships with others? Ability to function at work? Weight?"
- "What would be normal for you?"
- "What difficulties do you see in getting back to normal?"
- "What do you understand to be the cause of your condition?"
- "How do you intend to use the benefits of treatment?"

Specific treatment modalities selected should reflect:

- **Illness episode presenting for treatment** — Is the patient presenting with a manic, mixed, or depressive episode? The nature of the presenting episode plays a critical role in initiating treatment.
- **Severity** — Is the patient a danger to themselves or others? Is the patient a candidate for inpatient or intensive outpatient (day treatment) care?
- **Clinician readiness and scope of practice** — Does the clinician have the breadth and depth of knowledge necessary to treat the patient? Will the patient be referred immediately, transitioned to the specialty

mental health sector, or managed primarily in the primary care setting? Will consultation be required?

- **Patient readiness** — Is the patient adequately informed of the diagnosis and in agreement as to need for treatment and treatment strategy?

- **Quality of the therapeutic alliance** — Does the clinician possess the required empathy with the patient? Does the patient trust the clinician? Is there an agreement as to the need for treatment? Has the plan been discussed with the patient and any significant others?

- **Psychosocial considerations** — Does the patient have the support of significant others? Does the patient have his or her employer's support? Will a period of short-term disability be used? Is the appropriate paperwork available? Are there resources for psychotherapy, psychoeducation, and community support?

Concept of Mood Stabilizers

The classic definition of a "mood stabilizer" describes a psychotropic drug that improves both phases of the illness without worsening either phase and is effective in preventing new episodes. In addition, mood stabilizers do not exacerbate the maintenance phase of therapy.[3] Today, in addition to lithium, the term "mood stabilizer" is applied to certain anticonvulsant and atypical antipsychotic (AAP) drugs. Debate continues as to the most appropriate definition of a "mood stabilizer."

Using Treatment Guidelines

Pharmacologic interventions should proceed based on evidence-based guidelines. There are several published guidelines for the treatment of bipolar disorder. Such guidelines are products of both available evidence and the consensus of the expert panels convened to consider them. Several treatment guidelines reflect expert consensus, including:

Chapters 12 and 13 provide in-depth information on specific antimanic and antidepressant medications, including side effects and dosing guidelines.

- The American Psychiatric Association (APA) revised guideline published in 2002 (an update is planned for 2007)[4]
- The Canadian Network for Mood and Anxiety Treatments (CANMAT) published guidelines from 2005[5]
- An international consensus panel's guidelines for patients with bipolar I disorder[6]
- A guideline for the treatment of children and adolescents with bipolar disorder[7]
- The Texas Implementation of Medication Algorithm (TIMA) guidelines (see pages 156–157 and 161–163)[8]

The recommendations for treatment throughout this chapter are a compilation of TIMA and APA guidelines, unless otherwise noted.[4, 8] TIMA's recently revised, evidence-based algorithms reflect consensus panel decisions made in May 2004, when a diverse group of academic psychiatrists and clinical psychopharmacology specialists met to review the newest available evidence for selecting treatments for bipolar disorder. Other members of the panel were Texas Department of State Health Services administrators as well as community mental health physicians, advocates, and consumers. The panel based its decisions on evidence from well-controlled studies (when available), employing a method similar to the one used by the Agency for Healthcare Research and Quality (AHRQ) to develop guidelines for treating depression.

The authors of the TIMA guidelines stress several important caveats to guide clinicians when treating patients with bipolar disorder, including these:[8]

Guidelines are a starting place for treatment; they need both to be adapted to individual response and tolerance in order to achieve stabilization and to be continually updated to incorporate knowledge from new, high-quality scientific studies.

- **Patients should be treated by the core algorithm**. There are two stand-alone algorithms: for patients presenting with manic/hypomanic/mixed episodes, and for patients presenting with depressive episodes.

- **The algorithms focus on the treatment of core symptoms**. The goals are symptom remission and return to a healthy, functional level.

- **The most well-tolerated form of a given medication is recommended**.

- **Adjunctive medications are not described, but they may be required for comorbid conditions or symptoms, such as anxiety**.

- **Treatment decisions progress through stages and are based on inadequate response to treatment or medication intolerance**. Early stages include monotherapy with widely used medications. Later stages involve more complex medication combinations, with an attendant greater risk of side effects and monitoring requirements.

- **Change medications with an overlap-and-taper strategy, unless medical necessity requires abrupt discontinuation**.

- **Severely ill patients should be evaluated more often (e.g., weekly) than patients who are less ill**. It may be appropriate, depending on symptom severity and patient history, to start at a later stage.

INTRODUCTION

PRESENTATION

CLINICAL PROCESS

PHARMACOTHERAPY

RESOURCES

- **All treatment decisions should be based on clinician judgment and patient treatment history.**

- **Short-term improvements may not represent a stable drug effect.** After a clinical plateau is reached, patients should be evaluated for at least two weeks until clinical stability is confirmed. If the patient is stable during the evaluation period, the clinician can proceed with the continuation phase of treatment.

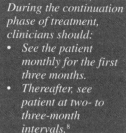

During the continuation phase of treatment, clinicians should:
- *See the patient monthly for the first three months.*
- *Thereafter, see patient at two- to three-month intervals.*[8]

The TIMA algorithms for bipolar I disorder were developed for both the patients presenting with acute depression (page 157) and the patient suffering with manic/hypomanic symptoms (page 162).

In the acute phase, the patient will most often present as depressed. If there has been a recent manic episode or a history of severe mania, initial treatment should include an anti-manic agent. Traditional antidepressant monotherapies should be discouraged as initial interventions, because they may worsen the acute or long-term course of the illness. Even when added to mood stabilizers for acute bipolar depression, antidepressants have limited efficacy and retain the potential for illness destabilization.[9] Mood stabilizers with evidence of efficacy in bipolar depression are preferred for initial drug treatment, and combinations of such agents may be used for persistent depressive symptoms.

In the maintenance phase, bipolar disorder should be treated as a highly recurrent illness. TIMA treatment recommendations for this phase appear on page 203 of chapter 11. Treatment selection for acute episodes should include consideration of ongoing maintenance treatment. Agents with evidence of both acute and maintenance efficacy may be preferred as long as no safety or tolerability obstacles exist.

Treating Bipolar I Disorder — Acute Bipolar Depression

Although various medications are used for treating acute bipolar depression, only quetiapine (an atypical antipsychotic) and an olanzapine-fluoxetine combination (an atypical antipsychotic plus an SSRI) are approved by the FDA for the acute treatment of bipolar depression. Lamotrigine monotherapy is indicated for patients **without** a history of severe and/or recent mania. For patients **with** a history of severe mania, lamotrigine should be used in combination with an antimanic medication.

Several issues complicate the decision to administer antidepressants. Prescribing antidepressants for patients with acute bipolar depression increases the risk of a mood switch (from depression to mania), although when used as add-on treatment, the risk is fairly low (5–12%).[10–15] Nevertheless, this type of drug must be administered only to depressed patients with bipolar I disorder who are also being treated with a mood stabilizer. Furthermore, depression must be carefully differentiated from dysphoric mania/hypomania or mixed symptoms and other more complicated states, since antidepressant monotherapy may simply unmask or exacerbate the mania.

Detailed discussion of the pharmacotherapy used in acute bipolar depression can be found in chapter 13.

Guidelines for selecting antidepressant therapy include:

- The severity of the patient's illness
- The presence or absence of psychotic manifestations
- The presence or absence of rapid cycling

TIMA Algorithm for Acute Depression

The TIMA strategy's algorithm for depression (figure 10.1 opposite page, describes these five stages of therapy:[8]

1. **Lamotrigine mono or combination therapy** — For patients **without** a history of severe and/or recent mania, lamotrigine (with or without lithium) is the initial therapeutic option. For patients on lithium with a history of severe and/or recent mania, optimize lithium dose (increase to ≥ 0.8 µEq/L). For all others, continue antimanic agent or add antimanic agent, and add lamotrigine.

2. **Quetiapine or olanzapine-fluoxetine combination (OFC)** — Both quetiapine monotherapy and the olanzapine-fluoxetine combination are FDA approved for bipolar depression.

3. **Combination therapy** — TIMA recommends choosing two from among lithium, lamotrigine, quetiapine, and OFC.

4. **Combination therapy including anti-depressants** — Broader choices for combination therapy exist and include antidepressants. Choose from lithium, lamotrigine, quetiapine, OFC, valproic acid/valproate, or carbamazepine plus an SSRI, bupropion, or venlafaxine; also, electroconvulsive therapy is an option.

5. **Other treatments** — Exploring remaining therapeutic options (e.g., MAOIs, tricyclic antidepressants, pramipexole, other atypical antipsychotics, oxcarbazepine, other combinations of drugs not previously listed, inositol, stimulants, thyroid supplementation).

MAOI therapy should be used cautiously because of the risk of severe hypertension due to dietary and drug interactions.

Figure 10.1   TIMA Algorithm: Acute BD I Depression

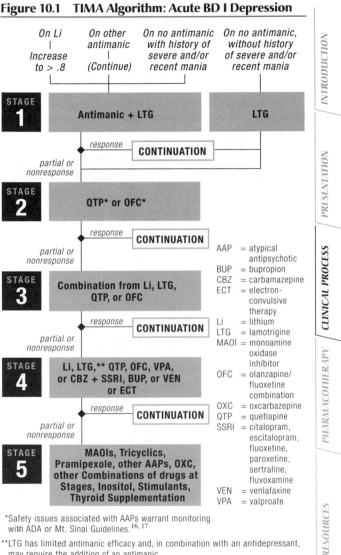

*Safety issues associated with AAPs warrant monitoring with ADA or Mt. Sinai Guidelines.[16, 17]

**LTG has limited antimanic efficacy and, in combination with an antidepressant, may require the addition of an antimanic.

Key Recommendations for Initial Approach to Therapy

The selection of initial therapy for the patient with acute bipolar depression should be based on the presenting manifestations. In addition, patient preferences should be considered whenever possible.

- Combination therapy may be more effective than monotherapy in patients with more severe illness.
- Psychotic manifestations are an indication to use or add an antipsychotic to the regimen.
- Antidepressant monotherapy is contraindicated in bipolar I disorder; however, quetiapine and an olanzapine-fluoxetine combination are FDA-approved therapeutic options.
- Electroconvulsive therapy (ECT) is a reasonable option for patients who are pregnant and severely depressed, suicidal, unwilling to eat or drink (to a life-threatening degree), or who are experiencing severe loss of vitality.
- After pharmacotherapy has been initiated, combination interpersonal therapy, cognitive behavioral therapy, or other psychotherapy may be useful once acute symptoms decrease.

BILL

Bill begins OFC treatment 6/25, one capsule daily in the early evening. He declined lithium because of previous bothersome side effects. In addition to being given printed and online reference information, Bill was cautioned about somnolence, asked to monitor his appetite, and informed that routine monitoring, including periodic blood glucose measurements, would be required.

Bill was referred to a psychotherapist for cognitive-behavioral therapy (CBT) and grief counseling. At a one-week follow-up visit, he was tolerating the medication well and reporting improved sleep and less sadness. Bill started paying more attention to his overall status and functioning and began addressing his grief and coping mechanisms.

At four weeks of therapy, he was "80 percent better" and the total score on his PHQ-9 had dropped from 24 to 10 (mild severity). He commented that "… everything was better except his level of energy and motivation, and insomnia was still a problem on some nights." Although he had no suicidal thoughts, residual symptoms included mild deficits in motivation; he related that it was "tough getting out of bed some days," and that he was low on energy – "just not my usual yet." In addition, Bill reported having occasional days when sadness was noticeable and when concentration on complex tasks like wiring buildings (he's an electrician) is a problem.

Key Recommendations for Breakthrough Episodes

• Optimize medical therapy.

• Obtain serum drug levels, especially when treatment involves lithium. If levels are not in range, increase doses until they are.

Key Recommendations for Inadequate Response

If a patient treated with combination therapy fails to show an adequate response and has therapeutic drug levels within the targeted range, several additional steps can be considered, including:[4]

• Reviewing the diagnosis to ensure that depressive manifestations are not secondary to a general medical disorder or drug/alcohol use

• Increasing medication dose(s) if side effects are tolerable

• Adding one of the newer antidepressants (e.g., venlafaxine) or an MAOI (e.g., tranylcypromine)

• Instituting add-on AAP if psychotic features are present

• Considering ECT if the patient is catatonic, fails to respond to above measures, has psychotic features, or is suicidal

Key Recommendations for Rapid Cycling

• Patients whose initial presentation includes rapid cycling should be treated with lithium, valproate, an atypical antipsychotic, or lamotrigine. If the patient is being treated with antidepressant monotherapy (due to unrecognized bipolar illness), the antidepressant dose should be tapered and the drug discontinued, if possible.

• Since rapid cycling may be caused or exacerbated by an associated general medical disorder (such as hypothyroidism or substance use), a detailed history (including medications and drugs) as well as appropriate lab tests should be obtained.

• If the patient is being treated with a mood stabilizer and an antidepressant, then combination regimens, possibly including an atypical antipsychotic, should be considered; tapering the antidepressant should be considered, as well.

Treating Bipolar I Disorder – Mania/Hypomania

The primary goals of therapy with antimanic agents are to rapidly control symptoms, such as agitation, impulsivity, and aggression, so that the patient can return to a normal level of functioning. Guidelines for selecting antimanic therapy are based on the severity of the patient's illness, the presence or absence of psychotic manifestations, and the presence or absence of rapid cycling.

Medications used to treat mania or hypomania include: lithium, anticonvulsants, atypical antipsychotics, and combination medications. Pages 167 through 179 provide an overview of the medications; see chapter 12 for detailed information.

TIMA Algorithm for Mania

The algorithm for treating those currently hypomanic/manic differentiates between treatment for those experiencing euphoric versus mixed symptoms. Additionally, it recommends targeted adjunctive treatment for those with acute symptoms, using clonidine or sedatives for agitated/aggressive symptoms, hypnotics for insomnia, and benzodiazepines or gabapentin for anxiety.

The TIMA algorithm for treatment of mania/hypomania (figure 10.2 on the next page) differentiates between entry points for patients experiencing euphoric symptoms or mixed symptoms. The algorithm describes these four stages of therapy:

1. **Monotherapy with a mood stabilizer** — Lithium is recommended only in cases of euphoric or irritable mania. Its efficacy in mixed episodes is less robust. The recommended first-line treatment in mixed-episode mania is a choice of valproate, aripiprazole, risperidone, or ziprasidone. The divalproex form of valproate is usually recommended because of its more favorable side-effect profile and tolerability. In addition to lithium, choices for treating euphoric or irritable mania include the agents above or quetiapine.

   In patients who demonstrate a partial response to optimum levels of a single mood stabilizer, the TIMA recommendation is to add a second agent (move to stage 2). However, patients who cannot tolerate the first single agent should be switched to another drug; choices include one of the above or alternates, such as olanzapine or carbamazepine. When possible, switching to another drug should be done through the overlap-and-taper method, unless it is medically necessary to discontinue a medication abruptly.

Figure 10.2   TIMA Algorithm: BD I Mania/Hypomania

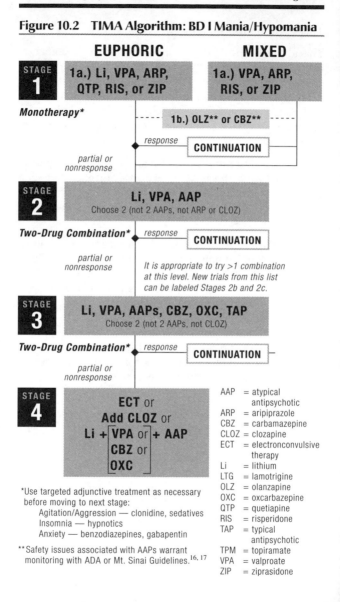

2. **Combination therapy** — This is standard care in most patients with bipolar mania. Choices include lithium, quetiapine, valproate, olanzapine, risperidone, and ziprasidone. The suggested combinations include lithium plus valproate, or lithium or valproate plus an AAP. More severely ill patients should start treatment at stage 2 instead of stage 1.

3. **Also combination therapy** — Compared with stage 2, there is a wider choice of drugs in stage 3, including aripiprazole, carbamazepine, and oxcarbazepine. If control of the illness is not achieved, advance to the next stage.

4. **Electroconvulsive therapy (ECT), clozapine, or three-drug combination** — The three-drug combination includes lithium, an anticonvulsant (valproate, carbamazepine, or oxcarbazepine), and an AAP.

The inclusion of olanzapine as a first-line agent was based on completed, well-controlled trials.[8] While olanzapine is listed as monotherapy for acute mania, the medication's side-effect profile and those of the other atypical antipsychotics should be considered before any member of this class is selected as first-line therapy. However, these agents now have FDA approval for use in acute mania.

Key Recommendations for Initial Approach to Therapy

• Prefer AAPs to typical antipsychotics because of the superior side-effect profile of AAPs.

• Discontinue antidepressants during treatment of acute mania.

• Combine pharmacotherapy with psychosocial therapy as the patient improves.

INTRODUCTION

PRESENTATION

CLINICAL PROCESS

PHARMACOTHERAPY

RESOURCES

Key Recommendations for Breakthrough Episodes

As with breakthrough episodes of acute depression (see page 159), checking serum levels and optimizing current therapy should be the first steps for patients presenting with acute mania or a mixed episode.[4]

- If medication levels are within target range, an AAP may be considered.

- Antipsychotics are also suggested when psychotic manifestations are present.

- Short-term treatment with a benzodiazepine can be used to decrease agitation, anxiety, and insomnia.

JANICE

Janice was evaluated and admitted for inpatient care. Her divalproex ER dose was titrated to therapeutic plasma levels. Olanzapine was continued at a dose of 15 mg daily. Janice was informed that blood testing would continue to be used to ensure proper dosing of the divalproex ER and to monitor various clinical parameters (liver function, platelet counts, glucose, and lipids). She was assured that adverse effects were relatively uncommon. Further, she was told that some sedation effect is common, principally early in treatment, and that she should report cognitive problems (memory or concentration), if experienced. Again, she was assured that most of these could be overcome with time and dose adjustment. Her psychoeducation included the rationale of using two medications at once to speed stabilization and remission of symptoms.

Janice recovered over a period of two months and returned to work. Her moods became predictable and even. She was much less easily angered and felt "in control" of her emotions. She found that she could be appropriately happy, sad, angry, or anxious, but she did not feel driven by her emotions beyond her abilities to think, act, and react appropriately.

Key Recommendations for Inadequate Response

With optimized, first-line mood stabilizers, manic symptoms should diminish within 10 to 14 days.[4] If treatment fails:

- Add carbamazepine or an AAP. If the regimen currently includes an AAP, substitute an alternative medication. For example, clozapine may be particularly effective in this situation for treatment-resistant patients.

- Confirm the diagnosis to ensure that clinical symptoms are not primarily due to a medical disorder or drug/alcohol substance use.

- Consider electroconvulsive therapy (ECT) for patients who are severely ill, resistant to pharmacotherapy, experiencing mixed episodes, pregnant, or who preferentially select ECT.

Treating Bipolar II Disorder and Cyclothymia

Bipolar II disorder is characterized by a greater number of episodes of major depression than bipolar I disorder, and has less frequent episodes of hypomania or mixed symptoms. For that reason, the focus of treatment in general should be on treating depression without destabilizing mood or inducing hypomania. Few controlled treatment studies focusing on bipolar II disorder have been completed, so general practice is to apply treatment recommendations for bipolar I disorder to bipolar II disorder.[4, 18] However, no evidence exists that the best options for bipolar I disorder are also best for bipolar II disorder.

Despite a general lack of research on treatment of bipolar II disorder, two well-controlled trials with significant sub-group analyses of bipolar II disorder have been completed for quetiapine and lamotrigine. Quetiapine was shown to be effective in the treatment of acute bipolar II depression, and lamotrigine was shown to be an effective maintenance treatment for bipolar II depression.[19, 20] Small, open label studies have been done to inform other treatment choices

Sidebar tabs (right margin): INTRODUCTION · PRESENTATION · CLINICAL PROCESS · PHARMACOTHERAPY · RESOURCES

for bipolar II disorder.[1, 18, 21] Several studies support the use of antidepressants in combination with mood stabilizers with a low risk of mood switch for both acute treatment and relapse prevention. Lithium also has several older studies supporting its use in the maintenance treatment of bipolar II. Further controlled studies are needed to more clearly define the best treatment options for bipolar II disorder.

HOLLY

Holly was encouraged to contact a psychotherapist, and received several names with contact numbers of therapists with a special interest in the psychoeducation and psychotherapy of patients with bipolar disorder. Holly was also asked to begin a walking program, starting with 30 minutes of brisk daily walking.

Having failed multiple antidepressant trials in the past, another trial of antidepressant monotherapy is not a consideration in her case. A complete metabolic panel, complete blood count, urinalysis, and TSH were within normal limits. Based on the American Psychiatric Association guidelines, Holly began treatment with lamotrigine (Lamictal) 25 mg daily for 2 weeks, then 50 mg daily for 2 weeks, then 100 mg daily for one week, and finally 200 mg QD. She was cautioned to report any unexpected rash immediately.

Holly reported modest improvement; she was less sad, had better motivation, and was less moody during her third week of lamotrigine. She achieved a robust remission with only minor, non-impairing symptoms (and only while under stressful circumstances). Holly's GAF (Global Assessment of Functioning) scores were usually greater than 80 (on a scale of 1–100, where higher scores mean better mental health). At the end of three months' therapy, she commented, "I don't think I've felt this well ever. Maybe this is what normal is supposed to be."

Cyclothymia is often a pre-bipolar II presentation. Attention should focus on mood stabilization in general, perhaps by starting with lithium or lamotrigine and moving to divalproex or an AAP, if needed. More research is needed in this area. Of note, however, preliminary data from a recent study by Kochman et al. showed that depressed children and adolescents with cyclothymic hypersensitive temperament were more likely to develop bipolar disorder than their cohorts without this particular temperament.[22]

Overview of Medication Treatments

Those medications approved by the FDA for treatment of acute mania or acute bipolar depression and for maintenance treatment appear in figure 10.3, below.

Figure 10.3   FDA-Approved Medications for Bipolar Treatment

Approved for Treating Acute Mania	Approved for Treating Acute Bipolar Depression
Medication (Trade Name)	**Medication (Trade Name)**
• Lithium (Lithobid®) • Chlorpromazine (Thorazine®) • Divalproex (Depakote®) • Olanzapine (Zyprexa®)* • Risperidone (Risperdal®)* • Quetiapine (Seroquel®)* • Ziprasidone (Geodon®) • Aripiprazole (Abilify®) • Carbamazepine (Equetro®)	• Olanzapine-fluoxetine combination (Symbyax®) • Quetiapine (Seroquel®)
Approved for Maintenance Treatment	
Medication (Trade Name)	
• Lithium (Lithobid®) • Lamotrigine (Lamictal®)	• Olanzapine (Zyprexa®) • Aripiprazole (Abilify®)

*Adjunctive, as well as monotherapy, use

These key medications have been studied extensively in recent clinical trials. Figure 10.4, on the next page, shows common trade names for those medications associated with bipolar treatment.

INTRODUCTION

PRESENTATION

CLINICAL PROCESS

PHARMACOTHERAPY

RESOURCES

Figure 10.4 Bipolar Medications/Trade Names

Common Medication and Trade Name(s)

- Lithium: Eskalith,® Lithobid®

Anticonvulsants

- Carbamazepine: Equetro,™ Tegretol,® Carbatrol®
- Gabapentin: Neurontin®
- Lamotrigine: Lamictal®
- Topiramate: Topamax®
- Valproate, divalproex, valproic acid: Depakote,® Depakene®

Antidepressants

- Amitriptyline: Elavil,® Endep®
- Amoxapine: Ascendin®
- Bupropion: Wellbutrin®
- Citalopram: Celexa®
- Clomipramine: Anafranil®
- Desipramine: Norpramin®
- Doxepin: Adapin,® Sinequan®
- Duloxetine: Cymbalta®
- Fluoxetine: Prozac®
- Fluvoxamine: Luvox®
- Imipramine: Tofranil®
- Maprotiline: Ludiomil®
- Mirtazapine: Remeron®
- Nortriptyline: Aventyl,® Pamelor®
- Paroxetine: Paxil®
- Protriptyline: Vivactil®
- Sertraline: Zoloft®
- Trazodone: Desyrel®
- Trimipramine: Surmontil®
- Venlafaxine: Effexor®

Atypical Antipsychotics (AAPs)

- Aripiprazole: Abilify®
- Clozapine: Clozaril,® FazaClo®
- Olanzapine: Zyprexa®
- Quetiapine: Seroquel®
- Risperidone: Risperdal®
- Ziprasidone: Geodon®

Combination Medications

- Olanzapine-Fluoxetine Combination: Symbyax®

Monoamine Oxidase Inhibitors (MAOIs)

- Isocarboxazid: Marplan®
- Phenelzine: Nardil®
- Selegiline: Eldepryl®
- Selegiline transdermal: Ensam®
- Tranylcypromine: Parnate®

Figure 10.5 Bipolar Disorder: Summary of Efficacy Evidence from Recent Clinical Trials (RCTs), below, compares results by drug for treating mania, depression, and ongoing maintenance. Specific information on clinical trials is included with the relevant sections of section D, chapters 12–14.

Figure 10.5 Bipolar Disorder: Summary of Efficacy Evidence from Recent Clinical Trials[23]

Medication	Mania Monotherapy	Mania Combination Therapy	Depression	Maintenance
Lithium	++	++*	+*	++
Divalproex	++	++*	+/–*	+/–*
Carbamazepine	++	ND*	+/–*	+/–*
Lamotrigine	–*	ND*	+*	++
Clozapine	ND*	ND*	ND*	+*
Olanzapine	++	++	++**	++
Risperidone	++	++	+/-*	ND*
Quetiapine	++	++	++	ND*
Ziprasidone	++	+*	ND*	ND*
Aripiprazole	++	ND*	ND*	+

++ = Two adequately powered trials with positive findings
+ = One adequately powered trial with positive findings
+/– = One adequately powered trial with equivocal findings
– = One adequately powered trial with negative findings
ND = No data

* Not FDA approved for this condition.

** Strongest evidence when taken in combination with fluoxetine; this combination is FDA approved for treating acute bipolar depression.

INTRODUCTION

PRESENTATION

CLINICAL PROCESS

PHARMACOTHERAPY

RESOURCES

The following brief overview covers medications used for treating bipolar disorder, including: lithium, anti-convulsants, antipsychotics (both typical and atypical), and antidepressants. Also discussed are combination and adjunctive therapies. Detailed information for these medications (and classes of medications) can be found in section D, chapters 12–14, organized according to their use as antimanic agents, antidepressants, or maintenance therapy. Those chapters cover clinical trial results, pharmacology, side effects, and administration.

Lithium

In 1970, lithium became the first drug to receive approval for the treatment of manic episodes in bipolar disorder.

See page 224 in chapter 12 and the Physicians' Desk Reference *for a comprehensive list of drugs affecting serum lithium levels.*

Since that time, it has become a mainstay of treatment for patients with acute mania. Lithium also has an FDA indication for maintenance treatment for preventing new episodes. Lithium's potential efficacy in the treatment of mania was first reported in 1949; however, concerns about the known potential effects of lithium toxicity restrained American psychiatrists from using it extensively until approved by the FDA in 1970.[24] Many drugs can alter serum lithium levels; some can mask gastrointestinal symptoms of lithium toxicity. Therefore, it is imperative that patients have their serum lithium levels monitored regularly.

Anticonvulsants

A number of research results indicate that certain anti-convulsant medications (e.g., divalproex, lamotrigine, carbamazapine) are helpful for treating mania and/or mixed states.

Divalproex/valproate/valproic acid (FDA-approved treatment for mania and mixed episodes) are variations of a simple, branched-chain carboxylic acid. This drug's anticonvulsant properties were discovered when it was used as a vehicle for drugs being screened for antiepileptic activity.

Lamotrigine (FDA approved as a maintenance treatment for prevention of new bipolar mood episodes) is particularly effective in decreasing the likelihood of new depressive episodes. The drug has a rare, potential side effect of medically serious rashes (Stevens Johnson Syndrome or toxic epidermal necrolysis). This risk is strongly associated with absolute starting dose and/or rate of initial titration. Thus, following the recommended medication-dosing schedule is critical.

Carbamazepine extended release (FDA-approved treatment for mania and mixed episodes) is chemically related to the tricyclic antidepressants. Although initially approved for the treatment of seizures, it has also been used to treat patients with various pain syndromes, such as trigeminal neuralgia. The drug has been used in combination with lithium for many years in Europe for treating acute mania; however, large, placebo-controlled, randomized clinical trials have only recently been completed with the extended-release formulation.[23] Carbamazepine has been shown to have antimanic activity in some patients who are refractory to lithium.

For TIMA 2005, the consensus panel placed carbamazepine as an alternate choice (stage 1b) despite adequate evidence of its efficacy due to concerns over drug interaction and tolerability.[8] These concerns can be addressed through careful management, such as monitoring blood levels and consideration of drug interactions; however, therapeutic blood levels are not required for carbamazepine ER.

Oxcarbazepine, which is structurally similar to carbamazepine, is pharmacologically a different drug, and direct tests of its efficacy in bipolar disorder are needed. This agent has been studied in open, uncontrolled trials; however, there is **no current FDA indication for bipolar**

disorder. It increases plasma levels of valproate and its metabolites are generally nontoxic. TIMA 2005 recommends oxcarbazepine as a stage-three medication (due to the lack of controlled studies) to be given in combination with those recommended for stage three.[8]

A number of other anticonvulsants have been studied as potential antimanic agents; however, studies of these drugs have been limited by sample size and methodologic issues. Of note, placebo-controlled studies with lamotrigine and topiramate in acute bipolar mania were negative.[2]

Typical Antipsychotics

Typical antipsychotics include haloperidol, chlorpromazine, thioridazine, and perphenazine. These medications have antimanic efficacy, particularly in patients with significant agitation.[25] However, their side effects limit their long-term use. These side effects include increased risk of depression, prolactin elevation, and extrapyramidal manifestations, such as tardive dyskinesia in patients with bipolar disorder. Therefore, they have been largely supplanted by the atypical antipsychotics.

Atypical Antipsychotics (AAPs)

Atypical antipsychotic agents are the newest additions to the psychotropic classes and are remarkable for their overall improved side-effect profile. However, patients treated with AAPs are still at risk for extrapyramidal side effects: akathisia, tardive dyskinesia, and neuroleptic malignant syndrome. The degree of this risk has not yet been fully defined and may vary across the agents in this class.

Several AAPs show beneficial effects in the treatment of depressive symptoms.

In 2005, the FDA issued a warning citing an increased risk of death in elderly patients treated with AAPs for dementia-related psychosis (not an indicated use for this medication).

Characteristics of these newer generation psychotropics include minimal-to-no extrapyramidal side effects and intrinsic antimanic properties. Other characteristics are discussed in chapter 12.

AAPs share many pharmacodynamic and pharmacokinetic properties, although they all have different adverse effects. Chief among these adverse effects are concerns about weight gain and increased risk of metabolic disorders.

The FDA issued a class warning for atypical antipsychotics regarding metabolic/diabetic issues in 2004. All patients receiving AAPs should be monitored for glycemic control issues and other metabolic effects (e.g., lipid and weight changes). At the present time, retrospective and prospective studies seem to differ on how strong this effect might be. Because atypical antipsychotics show great promise as efficacious agents in the treatment of bipolar disorder, a balanced, prudent approach should include accurate risk assessment prior to beginning therapy, including assessment of these questions:

1. Is there existing evidence of glycemic control abnormalities [e.g., prediabetic fasting plasma glucose (fpg) levels or frank diabetes mellitus, as evidenced by fpg or an abnormal oral glucose tolerance test (OGTT)]?
2. Is metabolic syndrome present? Does the patient have three of these five symptoms?[26]
   - Waist circumference greater than 40 inches (men) or 35 inches (women)
   - Triglyceride level > 150 mg/dL or being treated for high levels
   - HDL < 40 (men) or < 50 (women) or on medication for problem HDL

Based on the prospective data available, the absolute risk of treatment-emergent diabetes may be small relative to the benefit derived from treatment with AAPs.

- Blood pressure > 130/85 mm Hg or on antihypertensive medication
- FPG > 100 mg/dL or on medication for elevated blood glucose levels[27]

3. Is there a first-degree relative with type 2 diabetes mellitus (T2DM)?

4. Has the patient already been diagnosed with T2DM? Such patients may be at greatest risk of worsening glycemic control from the use of atypical antipsychotics. Therefore, the highest levels of glucose monitoring should be targeted at this group. When equivalent efficacy can be expected from agents lacking the potential for worsening glycemic control, these agents should be considered first when managing patients with comorbid T2DM. Self-monitored blood glucose (SMBG) testing may be appropriate, and patients can be instructed in its proper use. Careful attention to lifestyle and optimization of the existing medical management of diabetes is indicated.

> *Treatment recommendations for metabolic syndrome published by the National Cholesterol Education Project (NCEP) and the American Diabetes Association/American Psychiatric Association (ADA/APA) include:[16, 26, 28]*
>
> - *Therapeutic lifestyle changes involving diet, nutrition, and exercise*
> - *Regular follow-up monitoring*
> - *Consideration of switching antipsychotic medication for those who gain ≥ 5% of baseline body weight while taking a specific medication*

ADA guidelines should be used for monitoring all patients taking atypical antipsychotics.[16] At the 2004 Consensus Development Conference on Antipsychotic Drugs and Obesity and Diabetes, experts from the American Diabetes Association, American Psychiatric Association, Association of Clinical Endocrinologists, and the North American Association for the Study of Obesity proposed a monitoring protocol for patients taking atypical antipsychotic medications. Figure 10.6, below, illustrates that protocol.[16]

The ADA recommended pre-treatment assessment of risk and periodic monitoring with an fpg test at three months of treatment.[16] Patients with multiple risk factors (obesity, metabolic syndrome, family history, prediabetic fpg) warrant the next higher level of clinical monitoring. Clinicians may elect to institute more frequent monitoring earlier. Not all AAPs may carry the same metabolic risks; this is an area under very active study.

Figure 10.6   Monitoring Protocol for Patients Taking Atypical Antipsychotics*[16]

Screening Measures	Baseline	4 Weeks	8 Weeks	12 Weeks	Quarterly	Annually	Every 5 Yrs
Personal/family history	X					X	
Weight (BMI)	X	X	X	X	X		
Waist circumference	X			X		X	
Blood pressure	X			X		X	
Fasting plasma glucose (fpg)	X			X		X	
Fasting lipid profile	X			X			X

* More frequent assessments may be warranted if clinical status indicates need. (from American Diabetes Association et al., 2004).

Patients without significant pre-treatment diabetic risk may be at the lowest risk of treatment-emergent hyperglycemia/T2DM. Monitoring during treatment is recommended according to the ADA consensus guidelines.

Some atypical antipsychotics appear to have mood stabilizing properties; therefore, as a class, they might be anticipated to have efficacy in patients with acute bipolar depression. However, only quetiapine and an olanzapine-fluoxetine combination are currently approved by the FDA for treating

The only medications currently FDA approved for bipolar depression are quetiapine and an olanzapine-fluoxetine combination. Refer to prescribing information for FDA warnings on treating elderly patients with AAPs and on the risk of suicide in children and adolescents treated with antidepressants.

bipolar depression. Other atypical antipsychotics (to date) are being studied in randomized, controlled trials with patients suffering from acute bipolar depression. The relative impact that different members of this medication class might have on bipolar depression should soon be known.

Antidepressants

In 2005, the FDA required all antidepressants to carry a warning regarding the increased risk of suicide, especially in children and adolescents, in patients treated with this class of medications. Patients should be closely watched for any increase in suicide ideation while taking antidepressants.

As mentioned earlier in this chapter, prescribing antidepressants carries some risk of inducing a mood switch in a

Balancing mood stabilizers (antimanic and antidepressant agents) combined in a patient's treatment plan must be done on a case-by-case basis, weighing the relative risks and benefits for each patient.

patient with bipolar disorder. In addition, patients need to be aware that virtually all medications used to treat depression will require two to three weeks to bring about symptom improvement. Often those around the individual experiencing depression will see improvement before the patient does. Antidepressants are generally started after remission of manic symptoms if depression develops, or if a patient was euthymic (not manic or depressed) and develops new depressive symptoms. If a person is experiencing mood instability or rapid cycling, use of antidepressants may actually worsen or prolong the period of instability.

Antidepressants used in addition to antimanic agents for treating bipolar disorder include selective serotonin reuptake inhibitors (SSRIs), tricyclics (TCAs), bupropion, venlafaxine, duloxetine, and monoamine oxidase inhibitors (MAOIs).

SSRIs

SSRI medications, which enhance serotonergic transmission, are in widespread clinical use and are administered as a single daily dose (potentially enhancing compliance). SSRIs are commonly prescribed antidepressants that have efficacy in patients with both unipolar and bipolar depression. They are preferred to MAOIs and TCAs in many situations because of their tolerability and favorable side-effect profile. However, like other antidepressants, the SSRIs must be administered in conjunction with a mood stabilizer to prevent mood switches and cycle acceleration in patients with acute bipolar depression.

TCAs

Before the SSRIs and other alternative antidepressants were introduced, a TCA was the add-on drug of choice for the treatment of acute bipolar depression. However, TCAs are now generally considered second- or third-line agents for this indication.

Bupropion

Bupropion is an aminoketone antidepressant chemically unrelated to other antidepressants. Although its exact mechanism of action is not precisely known, bupropion inhibits the neuronal uptake of both dopamine and norepinephrine. Experimentally, the drug acts as a mild stimulant and can cause seizures in large doses. The drug is rapidly absorbed after administration, is metabolized and activated in the liver, and is excreted in the urine.

Bupropion has little side-effect impact on sexual functioning, relatively few drug interactions, and reasonable tolerability.

Venlafaxine

Venlafaxine is an antidepressant that enhances both nor-adrenergic and serotonergic neurotransmitters and belongs to class of antidepressants called serotonin-norepinephrine reuptake inhibitors (SNRIs). It works by blocking the transporter "reuptake" proteins for key neurotransmitters affecting mood. At low (37.5–75 mg) daily dosages, venlafaxine may inhibit serotonin reuptake alone, similar to the action of an SSRI. At higher dosages (150–225 mg and above), venlafaxine inhibits the reuptake of norepinephrine and serotonin. At high dosages (starting around 300 mg), it inhibits dopamine reuptake in addition to serotonin and norepinephrine. However, the maximum approved daily dose of venlafaxine XR in the treatment of major depression is 225 mg. In recent clinical trials with patients suffering from bipolar depression where an antidepressant was added to a mood stabilizer for acute treatment, venlafaxine carried a greater risk of mood switch than did sertraline or bupropion.[29]

Duloxetine

Duloxetine is another SNRI that is currently approved for the treatment of major depression, generalized anxiety disorder, and diabetic peripheral neuropathic pain. Doses up to 120 mg daily have been studied in clinical trials with mild-to-moderate nausea lasting less than one week being the chief adverse event reported.

MAOIs

These antidepressant drugs inhibit the monoamine oxidase enzyme (found in the central nervous system, intestinal tract, and platelets), which is linked to norepinephrine, a neurotransmitter implicated in the development of depression. However, because of the potential risk of a hypertensive crisis (very high abrupt change in blood pressure) that can occur as a result of food or medication interactions with MAOIs, these agents are typically used only after other treatments have failed **and** when safety risks have been thoroughly evaluated.

Combination Therapy

Combination therapy typi-
cally includes selections of
medications from different
drug classes, most notably

Most patients with bipolar disorder typically need more than one medication to achieve mood stability.

lithium, anticonvulsants, and AAPs. Typically, published
algorithms for treatment of bipolar disorder have recommended trying a single medication first, and then, if needed,
combining medications.[9, 30–32]

Newer guidelines recommend starting with combination
medications for those whose symptoms are more severe.[8, 33]
Recent studies support hypotheses that the use of two medications to treat acute mania may increase the degree of response
for many patients in the first three weeks of treatment.

Adjunctive and Other Therapies

ECT is an accepted, effective treatment for acute mania and
for depression, whether in patients with bipolar or unipolar
disorder.[34, 35] However, safety, tolerability, and patient acceptance issues typically rank ECT behind pharmacological
approaches. Because of the range of medications now
available, ECT is typically reserved for:

- Patients unresponsive to or unable to take
  current medications
- Women who are pregnant
- Patients in acute danger of committing suicide
- Patients who suffer dangerous lack of food and fluid
  intake because of severe depressive symptoms

The response to this treatment is quite rapid, with striking
improvements seen often within one to two weeks.

In addition to ECT, less-invasive techniques are being explored, such as repetitive transcranial magnetic
stimulation (rTMS) and vagal nerve stimulation (VNS).
In rTMS, a magnetic field passes through the dorsolateral
prefrontal cortex. Hypoactivity in this area is associated

with depression; stimulation appears to increase metabolic activity and, theoretically, function. In VNS, a pacemaker is inserted and a wire wrapped around the vagus nerve in the neck; the wire is then stimulated by a small electrical current every few minutes. Why this is effective is unknown.

Other alternative therapies are currently being studied, including adjunctive treatments using fish oils (Omega 3), acupuncture, and mineral supplements. Although researchers anticipate new developments from these studies, caution should be exercised before embracing alternative or complementary approaches. For example, kava kava (an herb sometimes used to combat anxiety) has recently been associated with cases of liver failure.[36]

Factors Influencing Medication Strategies

Factors affecting medication strategies include:

- **Medication side effects** — Effects on weight and cognition, as well as on sedation, metabolic implications, hematologic/hepatic/renal injury, and allergic/toxic sequelae, should all be considered.

  Detailed information on side effects common to antimanic agents appears in chapter 12; for antidepressants, see chapter 13.

- **Reproductive issues (pregnancy, post-partum, lactation)** — Because many bipolar patients are women in their childbearing years, they will need information on the benefits and risks of treatment, including guidance about using reliable birth control to anticipate pregnancy in overall bipolar treatment planning and consider actions of drug interactions.

- **Comorbidity and treatment impacts** — Comorbid medical conditions (e.g., heart, renal, or hepatic disease) can influence treatment decisions. For comorbid psychiatric disorders, treatment during and after stabilization of the bipolar disorder may include addressing comorbid anxiety disorders, problems with substance use, eating disorders, or attention deficit disorder.

• **Cultural and age-associated considerations** — These considerations may significantly affect treatment selection and medication adherence.

Medication Side Effects

Drugs used to treat bipolar disorder can have serious side effects. Furthermore, medication adverse effects are a significant factor in poor treatment compliance. Treatment strategies could vary based on side-effect profiles and the specific patient's health and lifestyle realities. For example, when selecting an atypical antipsychotic, the physician would want to choose a medication with less weight gain side effects for lethargic and obese patients. In any case, patients need to understand the possible side effects and their significance before starting on any specific treatment.

Importantly, the risk/benefit ratio must always be considered. If the medication that allows the greatest mood stabilization causes significant side effects, its benefits will need to be balanced against the likelihood of ongoing destabilization and associated risks. Recognition of this is reflected in the TIMA guidelines where, for example, inclusion of clozapine (associated with ongoing blood work monitoring, weight gain, and other side effects) is at a lower level. Some patients may need this treatment to fully stabilize, which can make a significant difference in the quality of life for such individuals.

Reproductive Issues

About 50 percent of all pregnancies are unintended.[37] Since all psychotropic agents carry the potential for negative effects on the developing fetus, and symptomatic bipolar disorder may also have negative effects on the fetus and the mother, information on pregnancy-associated risks should be shared with all women of childbearing age. Maintaining a balance between benefits/risks of medication during pregnancy requires:

- Consistent, effective chart documentation
- Reviewing regularly updated information on risks associated with various agents
- Consultation or referral in specific instances

The American Academy of Pediatrics Committee on Drugs (2001) considered both valproate and carbamazepine as "usually compatible" with breast feeding.[38] Lithium, once regarded as contraindicated in nursing mothers, is now classified as "should be given to nursing mothers with caution." No psychotropic medications are known to be absolutely safe in breast feeding. Bottle feeding with formula is the obvious alternative unless a wet nurse is available. Another option is a mix of breast and formula feeding, with breast feeding during the period of time with lowest serum concentrations of medications (e.g., trough levels).

Another concern for patients with bipolar disorder who are pregnant or nursing is that interrupting therapy may precipitate a mood episode. Therefore, when the patient elects to become pregnant or has discovered that she is pregnant, the patient, partner, and clinicians (primary care, obstetrician, psychiatrist) must work together to assess the risks/benefits of various medication strategies.

It is important to note that valproate, a recommended antimanic treatment, appears to be associated with an increased risk of developing polycystic ovarian syndrome (PCOS). Joffe et al., in a recent retrospective study, found that incidence of women with bipolar disorder who developed PCOS while taking valproate was 10.5 percent, compared with 1.4 percent of women receiving non-valproate anticonvulsant or lithium.[39] This risk was particularly noted in younger women (≤ 25 years of age). While the rate of PCOS associated with valproate treatment was lower than previously reported, the possible long-term consequences of PCOS merit careful monitoring of female patients treated with this agent.

Comorbidity and Treatment Impacts

The presence of a comorbid medical or psychiatric condition can exacerbate bipolar disorder, just as bipolar disorder can exacerbate a medical condition. Note that diuretics, angiotensin-converting enzyme inhibitors, nonsteroidal anti-inflammatory drugs, and low-salt diets all alter the excretion of lithium.[4] Essential drugs that affect cardiac conduction and rhythm, or alter the function of organ systems involved in drug excretion, may all limit the choice of medication. HIV-infected patients with bipolar disorder are at increased risk of both drug-related adverse events (because of their altered immune status) and potential drug-to-drug interactions (created by the spectrum of drugs used to treat the infection and prevent complications).

Monitoring for potential drug interactions between medications for bipolar disorder and other conditions (as well as over-the-counter medications) is also an important issue in illness management.

In part because of medication side effects, patients with bipolar disorder are at greater risk for cardiovascular disease, cancer, obesity, and T2DM than is the general population. Meanwhile, patients with bipolar disorder are just as susceptible to these and other common medical illnesses as the general population. As discussed previously, the increased risk for obesity and T2DM, which can be exacerbated by weight gain from some bipolar disorder treatments, suggests that monitoring of body weight, calculation of body mass index (BMI), and education about sound diet, nutrition, and exercise are important components of treatment.[40] In addition, baseline and at least annual screening for hyperglycemia and dyslipidemias are important, especially in the presence of other risk factors for diabetes and metabolic syndrome (e.g., hypertension, family history of diabetes, age, ethnicity, physical inactivity). These are general recommendations regardless of the medication regimen of the patient.

For patients with bipolar disorder and comorbid psychiatric symptoms, the current approach recommended in all APA and national guidelines is to treat comorbid symptoms with recommended treatments following stabilization of bipolar symptoms. This is especially true when antidepressants or psychostimulants are under consideration for treatment of the comorbid condition. Special treatment considerations involve comorbid substance abuse and anxiety disorders as well as associated psychotic symptoms.

Substance Abuse

Comorbid substance abuse can significantly complicate therapy for patients with bipolar disorder. For example, inhibition of antidiuretic hormone by alcohol can predispose patients to dehydration and the potential for lithium toxicity. Chronic liver disease in patients with alcoholism

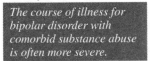

The course of illness for bipolar disorder with comorbid substance abuse is often more severe.

or chronic hepatitis C can alter the pharmacokinetics of valproate, carbamazepine, and other medications.

Though there are few studies, some evidence suggests that anticonvulsant mood stabilizers, such as divalproex and carbamazepine, may be better than lithium for populations of patients with comorbid substance abuse, and their use may also improve treatment compliance.[41, 42] Other studies suggest that increased patient contact, at the rate of up to two clinical contacts per week, as well as psychosocial support (group meetings and counseling), may also help improve patient outcomes and decrease hospitalizations and positive drug screens.[43]

Comorbid Anxiety Disorder

Anxiety disorders are among the most common comorbid conditions in patients with bipolar disorders.[44, 45] The prevalence of anxiety disorders in bipolar disorder varies widely among studies, depending on the sample, but all studies agree that patients with bipolar disorder and comorbid anxiety disorder have a poorer course of illness and lower response to treatment.[44, 46, 47]

The treatment of comorbid anxiety disorder in bipolar disorder presents a challenge to clinicians. In primary care settings, the presence of severe anxiety or panic states may be a significant distraction from a proper diagnosis of bipolar disorder. Establishing or excluding bipolar disorder is a foundational task in the assessment of the anxious patient. The most common method of treating anxiety disorders, usually using TCAs or SSRIs, can result in the development of mania or hypomania in bipolar patients.[48] Clinicians should first use mood stabilizers before cautiously beginning a treatment regimen for the anxiety disorder.[49]

Although lithium is commonly prescribed for bipolar disorder, a review of research suggests that valproate may sometimes be a good choice for comorbid anxiety, as it appears to improve symptoms in patients with panic disorder and OCD.[50] A recent review of atypical antipsychotic studies shows that these drugs, in addition to their mood stabilizing properties, also may have anxiolytic effects in patients with anxiety disorders, including OCD, PTSD, and GAD.[51] However, few published studies exist that directly examine the treatment of comorbid anxiety and bipolar disorders. Studies are currently underway to assess treatment for patients with bipolar and anxiety disorders.

Associated Psychotic Symptoms

Psychotic manifestations may occur during a manic episode. If mild, antipsychotic drugs may not be required, and lithium or another agent may be adequate. If severe, an atypical antipsychotic can be administered during the acute phase and continued during maintenance therapy. Approximately 20 to 30 percent of patients with bipolar mania may show catatonic symptoms, such as motor excitement, mutism, and stereotypic movements. Although ECT appears to be the most effective intervention in patients with catatonic features, lorazepam may also be effective and can be prescribed before other options are used.[52, 53]

Cultural and Age-Associated Concerns

Variations in drug metabolism related to race and ethnicity are cultural considerations that may affect drug dosage levels and responses. For example, Chinese patients have lower average activities of CYP2D6 and 2C9 than Caucasians. This is an area where too little is known and research to define any racial differences in response to treatment is ongoing.

Pharmacotherapy for **elderly patients** with bipolar disorder requires special care, because these patients have reduced dose requirements, alterations in drug pharmacokinetics associated with renal or hepatic disease, and higher risks for drug-induced cognitive impairment, and extrapyramidal side effects, such as tardive dyskinesia, orthostatic hypotension, and falls.[4]

Elderly patients may have increased end-organ sensitivity that increases both their response and the risk of side effects.

Age-associated changes in renal clearance and volume of distribution generally reduce the dose requirements for lithium and other psychoactive drugs in the elderly.[4, 54] Associated chronic renal or hepatic disease can also alter the pharmacokinetics of drugs used to treat patients with bipolar illness. However, in the absence of side effects or demonstrable efficacy in an elderly patient, the dose of the drug should be slowly increased until it is in the therapeutic range.

Multimodal Approaches and Their Efficacy

Bipolar disorder is a pervasive disorder requiring a mutimodal approach. Psychotherapy is recommended for all patients, particularly approaches that include structured psychoeducation, cognitive therapy, or other structured therapies. In addition, other biological treatments [i.e., electroconvulsive therapy (ECT), vagal nerve stimulation (VNS), and transcranial magnetic stimulation (rTMS)] show promise as adjunct therapies.

> *These approaches are primarily recommended during the stabilization and maintenance phases of treatment.*

Psychosocial Therapy

Both psychosocial therapy outcome studies and published treatment guidelines support the use of psychosocial treatment approaches as a possible adjunct to pharmacological therapy. Longitudinal data collected in the 1990s suggest that those with bipolar disorder suffer relapse at rates as high as 40 percent (year one), 60 percent (year two), and 73 percent (years 5+).[55] According to recent reviews of psychosocial therapy outcome studies in bipolar disorder, psychoeducational and cognitive-behavioral strategies (included as an adjunct to traditional pharmacological treatments) result in a decreased rate of hospitalization and incidence of relapse, as well as improved medication adherence and improved overall clinical symptoms.[55–57]

Published guidelines for treating bipolar disorder also support the use of psychosocial interventions.[3, 8, 16, 18] For example, the "Expert Consensus Guideline" for bipolar disorder endorses mood-stabilizing medication as the first line of treatment for depression in bipolar disorder, but includes alternative options of either treatment with an antidepressant medication or addition of psychosocial therapy to existing medication.[9]

Psychosocial interventions are appropriate measures to help the patient deal with disease-related issues, self-esteem,

INTRODUCTION

PRESENTATION

CLINICAL PROCESS

PHARMACOTHERAPY

RESOURCES

and adherence to treatment. They are especially useful in educating the patient about the disorder and combating misinformation, as well as in overcoming a patient's denial of illness. Psychosocial interventions are also very helpful in overcoming negative stigma (a sense of disgrace or moral blemish) that patients may have regarding a diagnosis of bipolar disorder; they help in setting behavioral boundaries that minimize risk-taking, allow proper sleep hygiene, and limit exposure to substances that may negatively affect mood. Social rhythm therapy, an approach derived from a chronobiological model of bipolar disorder, is an individual psychotherapy that combines interpersonal psychotherapy with attempts to encourage regular daily routines, address interpersonal problems and maximize medication adherence. Social rhythm therapy attempts to reduce disease effects on circadian and sleep-wake cycles and to improve function.[58]

Although focused psychosocial therapy may be effective in patients with acute bipolar depression, it fails to reduce manic symptoms, even when combined with pharmaco-therapy. Psychosocial treatments are particularly indicated when patients:

- Need help understanding and accepting the need for long-term pharmacotherapy
- Require an adjunct to pharmacotherapy as a stable component of the overall therapeutic regimen
- Refuse medications
- Want to avoid antidepressant-related adverse events (e.g., agitation or rapid cycling)
- Are being treated in the maintenance phase of bipolar illness

Figure 10.7, beginning on the next page, summarizes those psychosocial interventions proven effective as adjunctive therapy: psychoeducation; family focused treatment (FFT); and psychotherapy approaches, specifically interpersonal social rhythm therapy (IPSRT) and cognitive-behavioral therapy (CBT).

Figure 10.7 Psychosocial Interventions

Type	Objectives	Potential Strategies
Psychoeducational	• Teach patient and family members about the nature of the disorder and bipolar disorder management skills • Provide reading materials and videos supporting these topics	• Stress the importance of medication adherence • Identify potential precipitating factors • Recognize early relapse

Psychoeducational Efficacy Results

Study of 21 structured group sessions indicated:[59]
• Significantly reduced recurrences
• Increased time between episodes
• Decreased number and length of hospitalizations

Family Focused Treatment (FFT)	• Assist the patient with resolving interpersonal issues that may result from the illness or associated psychiatric comorbidities	• Participate in family or marital therapy to improve communications and problem solving between family members

FFT Efficacy Results

Studies of various approaches found:[60–62]
• Decreased relapse rates and hospitalization
• Increased relapse-free intervals
• Improved medication adherence
• More effective depression prevention and less severe depressive symptoms when relapse did occur

Psychotherapeutic (IPSRT and CBT)	• Help patients accept loss • Build self-image and confidence • Focus on maintaining stable life habits and managing stress	• Identify/reduce feelings of sadness or grief from loss of a loved one, a job, personal possessions, or inability to meet unrealistic goals • Achieve a healthy, realistic self-image • Establish consistent eating and sleeping schedules

(continued)

INTRODUCTION

PRESENTATION

CLINICAL PROCESS

PHARMACOTHERAPY

RESOURCES

Figure 10.7 (continued)

Type	Objectives	Potential Strategies
Psychotherapeutic Efficacy Results		

For IPSRT, intensive clinical management studies indicated:[58, 63, 64]
- Increased stability of daily routines and sleep/wake cycles
- Patients in IPSRT one year more likely to remain euthymic
- Consistency of intervention (1 regimen or the other) was associated with lower rates of relapse (20% vs. 40%) > 1 year*
- Failure to produce an additive benefit on relief of depressive symptoms or time to remission

For CBT, studies found:[65–68]
- Improved medication adherence
- Decreased mood disorder hospitalizations
- Enhanced self-identification of early mood symptoms and earlier medical intervention
- Reduced relapse rates
- Significantly improved social functioning over 18 months
- Reduced depressive symptoms (Adding CBT to mood-stabilizing pharmacotherapy was as effective as CBT alone for patients with unipolar depression)
- Improved global functioning

*Patients were re-randomized during the study; those randomized to continue in the same group had improved outcomes.

Electroconvulsive Therapy (ECT)

The use of ECT as maintenance therapy is appropriate for patients who have:[4]

- Been diagnosed as having refractory or severe acute bipolar mania or depression, particularly if psychotic features or suicidal ideations are also present
- Achieved remission of a major mood episode through ECT in the past

Controlled studies have demonstrated that ECT is superior to placebo and at least as effective as TCA or MAOI therapy.[34] ECT has been shown to produce outcomes superior to combination therapy with lithium and haloperidol.[34]

In addition, an older study found that patients treated with ECT followed by lithium maintenance therapy improved more than did patients treated with lithium alone during acute mania and in the maintenance phase.[35]

Vagal Nerve Stimulation

Vagal nerve stimulation (VNS) treatment involves implanting a small pulse generator in the chest that sends electrical signals into the brain via the vagus nerve. This non-pharmacologic biological treatment was approved in 1997 for treatment of refractory epilepsy. Recently, VNS was approved by the FDA for treatment-resistant depression.

Three recent studies found VNS to be effective for treatment-resistant depression.[69–71] One small pilot study has been completed in rapid cycling bipolar disorder with VNS, which also showed positive results. The study looked at 10 treatment-resistant adults with rapid-cycling bipolar disorder. Patients received VNS in addition to medication treatment for a year. All nine patients who were eligible to complete the study showed statistically significant improvement in severity of symptoms, as measured by the Life Charting Methodology (LCM). Statistically significant improvement was also seen in MADRS scores.[72]

Transcranial Magnetic Stimulation (rTMS)

This technique uses a coil placed against the scalp with an alternating current running through it, creating a powerful magnetic force that stimulates neurons in the brain. Evidence is mounting that rTMS may be quite helpful alone or in augmentation of psychotherapy and medication in the treatment of several refractory psychiatric conditions. Factors influencing its efficacy include whether left, right, or bilateral stimulation is used, the use of 80 percent vs. 100 percent of motor threshold stimulation, the length of treatment, and the cycle rate of stimulation (5 Hz vs. 10 Hz).[73]

Several trials show a statistical advantage to using rTMS, and the procedure is very well tolerated.[74–77] Substantial clinical benefit is still unproven, mostly because the studies were small, uncontrolled, and brief.[74–76, 78] Larger, multicenter studies should further clarify what role rTMS can play in the treatment of bipolar depression.[74] Of note, a 2002 meta-analysis by Kozel and George did find measurable clinical improvement when rTMS was used in the treatment of depression.[77] Saba et al., in an open case study that included psychotropic medication, also found benefits when rTMS was used to treat mania.[75]

References for Chapter 10

1. Suppes T, Dennehy EB. Evidence-based long-term treatment of bipolar II disorder. *J Clin Psychiatry*. 2002;63(Suppl 10)29–33.

2. American Psychiatric Association, American Psychiatric Association Task Force on DSM-IV. *Diagnostic and Statistical Manual of Mental Disorders: DSM-IV-TR*. Washington, DC: American Psychiatric Association; 2000.

3. Sachs GS. Bipolar mood disorder: practical strategies for acute and maintenance phase treatment. *J Clin Psychopharmacol*. 1996;16(Suppl 2):32S-47S.

4. American Psychiatric Association. Practice guideline for the treatment of patients with bipolar disorder (revision). *Am J Psychiatry*. 2002;159(Suppl 4):1–50.

5. Yatham LN, Kennedy SH, O'Donovan C, et al. Canadian Network for Mood and Anxiety Treatments (CANMAT) guidelines for the management of patients with bipolar disorder: consensus and controversies. *Bipolar Disord*. 2005;7(Suppl 3):5–69.

6. Kramer TA; for the International Consensus Group on Bipolar I Depression Treatment. International Consensus Group on Bipolar I Depression Treatment Guidelines: synopsis and discussion. *MedGenMed*. 2004 Apr;6(2):29.

7. Kowatch RA, Fristad M, Birmaher B. Treatment guidelines for children and adolescents with bipolar disorder. *J Am Acad Child Adolesc Psychiatry*. 2005;44(3):213–35.

8. Suppes T, Dennehy EB, Hirschfeld RM, et al. The Texas Implementation of Medication Algorithms: update to the algorithms for treatment of bipolar I disorder. *J Clin Psychiatry*. 2005;66(7):870–86.

9. Sachs GS, Printz DJ, Kahn DA, et al. The Expert Consensus Guideline Series: Medication Treatment of Bipolar Disorder 2000. *Postgrad Med*. 2000;Spec No:1–104.

10. Goodwin FK, Fireman B, Simon GE, et al. Suicide risk in Bipolar Disorder during treatment with lithium and divalproex. *JAMA*. 2003;290:1467–73.

11. Wehr TA, Goodwin FK. Can antidepressants cause mania and worsen the course of affective illness? *Am J Psychiatry*. 1987;144(11):1403–11.

12. Coryell W, Endicott J, Maser JD, et al. Long-term stability of polarity distinctions in the affective disorders. *Am J Psychiatry*. 1995;152(3):385–90.

13. Altshuler LL, Post RM, Leverich GS, et al. Antidepressant-induced mania and cycle acceleration: a controversy revisited. *Am J Psychiatry*. 1995;152(8):1130-8.

14. Nemeroff CB, Evans DL, Gyulai L, et al. Double-blind, placebo-controlled comparison of imipramine and paroxetine in the treatment of bipolar depression. *Am J Psychiatry*. 2001;158:906–12.

15. Post RM, Weiss SR. Sensitization and kindling phenomena in mood, anxiety, and obsessive-compulsive disorders: the role of serotonergic mechanisms in illness progression. *Biol Psychiatry*. 1998;44(3):193–206.

16. American Diabetes Association, American Psychiatric Association, American Association of Clinical Endocrinologists, et al. Consensus development conference on antipsychotic drugs and obesity and diabetes. *Diabetes Care*. 2004;27:596–601.

17. Marder SR, Essock SM, Miller AL, et al. Physical health monitoring of patients with schizphrenia. *Am J Psychiatry*. 204;161:1334–49.

18. Yatham LN. Diagnosis and management of patients with bipolar II disorder. *J Clin Psychiatry*. 2005;66(Suppl 1):13–7.

19. Hirschfeld RM, Suppes T, Vieta E, et al. *Quetiapine Monotherapy is Efficacious for Depressive Episodes in Patients with Bipolar II Disorder.* Presented at the 159th Annual Meeting of the American Psychiatric Association, Toronto, Canada, NR277; May 20-25, 2006.

20. Calabrese JR, Suppes T, Bowden CL, et al; for the Lamictal 614 Study Group. A double-blind, placebo-controlled, prophylaxis study of lamotrigine in rapid-cycling bipolar disorder. *J Clin Psychiatry*. 2000;61:841–50.

21. MacQueen GM, Young LT. Bipolar II disorder: symptoms, course, and response to treatment. *Psychiat Serv*. 2001;52(1):358–61.

22. Kochman, FJ, Hantouchec EG, Ferrari P, et al. Cyclothymic temperament as a prospective predictor of bipolarity and suicidality in children and adolescents with major depressive disorder. *Journal of Affective Disorders*. 2005;85:181–9.

23. Keck PE Jr, McElroy SL. Treatment of bipolar disorder. *Textbook of Psychopharmacology*. 3rd Edition. Nemeroff CB, Schatzberg AF, eds. American Psychiatric Publishing, Inc., Washington, DC, 2004.

24. Goodman LS, Hardman JG, Limbird LE, Gilman AG. *Goodman & Gilman's The Pharmalogical Basis of Therapeutics*. New York: McGraw Hill; 2001..

25. Moller HJ, Nasrallah HA. Treatment of bipolar disorder. *J Clin Psychiatry*. 2003;64 (Suppl 6):9-17; discussion 28.

26. National Cholesterol Education Program (NCEP) Expert Panel on Detection, Evaluation, and Treatment of High Blood Cholesterol in Adults(Adult Treatment Panel III). Third report of the NCEP panel on detection, evaluation, and treatment of high blood cholesterol in adults (adult treatment panel III). *Circulation*. 2002;106(25):3143–421.

27. Grundy SM, Cleeman JI, Daniels SR, et. al. Diagnosis and management of the metabolic syndrome: an American Heart Association/National Heart, Lung, and Blood Institute scientific statement: executive summary. *Circulation*. 2005;112:1–6.

28. American Diabetes Association. Screening for type 2 diabetes. *Diabetes Care*. 2004;27(Suppl 1):S11–14.

29. Leverich GS, Altshuler LL, Frye MA, et al. Risk of switch in mood polarity to hypomania or mania in patients with bipolar depression during acute and continuation trials of venlafaxine, sertraline, and bupropion as adjuncts to mood stabilizers. *Am J Psychiatry*. 2006;163:232–9.

30. Hirschfeld RM, Bowden DL, Gitlin MJ, et al. Practice guideline for the treatment of patients with bipolar disorder (revision). *Am J Psychiatry*. 2002;159 (Suppl):1-50.

31. Suppes T, Dennehy EB, Swann AC, et al; for the Texas Consensus Conference Panel on Medication Treatment of Bipolar Disorder. Report of the Texas Consensus Conference Panel on medication treatment of bipolar disorder 2000. *J Clin Psychiatry*. 2002;63(4):288–99.

32. Dennehy EB, Suppes T. Medication algorithms for bipolar disorder. *J Pract Psychiatry Behav Health*. 1999;5:142–52.

33. Keck PE Jr, Perlis RH, Otto MW, et al. The Expert Consensus Guideline Series: Treatment of Bipolar Disorder 2004. Postgrad Med. 2004;Spec Rep:1–120.

34. Mukherjee S, Sackeim HA, Schnurr DB. Electroconvulsive therapy of acute manic episode: a review of 50 years' experience. *Am J Psychiatry*. 1994;151(2):169-76.

35. Small JG, Klapper MH, Kellams JJ, et al. Electroconvulsive treatment compared with lithium in the management of manic states. *Arch Gen Psychiatry*. 1988;45(8):727–32.

36. Ernst E. Safety concerns about kava. *Lancet*. 2002;359:1865.

37. Finer L, Henshaw S. Disparities in rates of unintended pregnancy in the United States, 1994 and 2001. *Perspectives on Sexual and Reproductive Health*. 2006;38(2):90-6.

38. Committee on Drugs. American Academy of Pediatrics. Use of psychoactive medication during pregnancy and possible effects on the fetus and newborn. *Pediatrics*. 2000;105(4 Pt 1):880–7.

39. Joffe H, Cohen LS, Suppes T, et al. Valproate is associated with new-onset oligoamenorrhea with hyperandrogenism in women with bipolar disorder. *Biol Psychiatry*. 2006;59:1078–86.

40. Citrome L, Jaffe A, Levine J, et al. Relationship between antipsychotic medication treatment and new cases of diabetes among psychiatric inpatients. *Psychiatr Serv*. 2004;55(9):1006–13.

41. Goldberg JF, Garno JL, Leon AC, et al. A history of substance abuse complicates remission from acute mania in bipolar disorder. *J Clin Psychiatry*. 1999;60(11):733-40.

42. Weiss RD, Greenfield SF, Najavits LM, et al. Medication compliance among patients with bipolar disorder and substance use disorders. *J Clin Psychiatry*. 1998;59:172–4.

43. Sloan KL, Rowe G. Substance abuse and psychiatric illness: treatment experience. *Am J Drug Alcohol Abuse*. 1998;24:589–601.

44. Keck PE Jr, Strawn JR, McElroy SL. Pharmacologic treatment considerations in co-occurring bipolar and anxiety disorders. *J Clin Psychiatry*. 2006;67(Suppl 1):8–15.

45. McElroy SL. Diagnosing and treating comorbid (complicated) bipolar disorder. *J Clin Psychiatry*. 2004;65(Suppl 15):35–44.

46. Gaudiano BA, Miller IW. Anxiety disorder comorbidity in bipolar I disorder: relationship to depression severity and treatment outcome. *Depress Anxiety*. 2005;21:71–7.

47. Henry C, van den Bulke D, Bellivier F, et al. Anxiety disorder in 318 bipolar patients: prevalence and impact on illness severity and response to mood stabilizer. *J Clin Psychiatry*. 2003;64:331–5.

48. Perugi G, Toni C, Frare F, et al. Obsessive-compulsive-bipolar comorbidity: a systematic exploration of clinical features and treatment outcome. *J Clin Psychiatry*. 2002;63:1129–34.

49. Sasson Y, Chopra M, Harrari E, et al. Bipolar comorbidity: from diagnostic dilemmas to therapeutic challenge. *Int J Neuropsychopharmacol*. 2003;6(2):139–44.

50. Freeman MP, Freeman SA, McElroy SL. The comorbidity of bipolar and anxiety disorders: prevalence, psychobiology, and treatment issues. *J Affective Disorders*. 2002;68:1–23.

51. McIntyre R, Katzman M. The role of atypical antipsychotics in bipolar depression and anxiety disorders. *Bipolar Disord*. 2003;5(Suppl 2):20–35.

53. Hawkins JM, Archer KJ, Strakowski SM, et al. Somatic treatment of catatonia. *Int J Psychiatry Med*. 1995;25(4):345–69.

53. Bush G, Fink M, Petrides G, et al. Catatonia. II. Treatment with lorazepam and electroconvulsive therapy. *Acta Psychiatr Scand*. 1996;93(2):137–43.

54. Sproule BA, Hardy BG, Shulman KI. Differential pharmacokinetics of lithium in elderly patients. *Drugs Aging*. 2000;16(3):165–77.

INTRODUCTION

PRESENTATION

CLINICAL PROCESS

PHARMACOTHERAPY

RESOURCES

55. Otto MW, Reilly-Harrington N, Sachs GS. Psychoeducational and cognitive-behavioral strategies in the management of bipolar disorder. *J Affect Disord*. 2003;73(1-2):171–81.

56. Gonzalez-Pinto A, Gonzalez C, Enjuto S, et al. Psychoeducation and cognitive-behavioral therapy in bipolar disorder: an update. *Acta Psychiatr Scand*. 2004 Feb;109(2):83–90.

57. Swartz HA, Frank E. Psychotherapy for bipolar depression: a phase specific treatment strategy? *Bipolar Disord*. 2001;3:11–22.

58. Frank E, Swartz HA, Kupfer DJ. Interpersonal and social rhythm therapy: managing the chaos of bipolar disorder. *Biol Psychiatry*. 2000;48(6):593–604.

59. Colom F, Vieta E, Martinez-Aran A, et al. A randomized trial on the efficacy of group psychoeducation in the prophylaxis of recurrences in bipolar patients whose disease is in remission. *Arch Gen Psychiatry*. 2003;60(4):402–7.

60. Miklowitz DJ, Simoneau TL, George EL, et al. Family-focused treatment of bipolar disorder: 1-year effects of a psychoeducational program in conjunction with pharmacotherapy. *Biol Psychiatry*. 2000;48(6):582–92.

61. Rea MM, Tompson MC, Miklowitz DJ, et al. Family-focused treatment versus individual treatment for bipolar disorder: results of a randomized clinical trial. *J Consult Clin Psychol*. 2003;71(3):482–92.

62. Miklowitz DJ, George EL, Richards JA, et al. A randomized study of family-focused psychoeducation and pharmacotherapy in the outpatient management of bipolar disorder. *Arch Gen Psychiatry*. 2003;60(9):904–12.

63. Frank E, Swartz HA, Mallinger AG, et al. Adjunctive psychotherapy for bipolar disorder: effects of changing treatment modality. *J Abnorm Psychol*. 1999;108(4):579–87.

64. Cole DP, Thase ME, Mallinger AG, et al. Slower treatment response in bipolar depression predicted by lower pretreatment thyroid function. *Am J Psychiatry*. 2002;159(1):116–21.

65. Cochran SD. Preventing medical noncompliance in the outpatient treatment of bipolar affective disorders. *J Consult Clin Psychol*. 1984;52(5):873–8.

66. Perry A, Tarrier N, Morriss R, et al. Randomised controlled trial of efficacy of teaching patients with bipolar disorder to identify early symptoms of relapse and obtain treatment. *BMJ*. 1999;318(7177):149–53.

67. Scott J, Garland A, Moorhead S. A pilot study of cognitive therapy in bipolar disorders. *Psychol Med*. 2001;31(3):459–67.

68. Zaretsky AE, Segal ZV, Gemar M. Cognitive therapy for bipolar depression: a pilot study. *Can J Psychiatry*. 1999;44(5):491–4.

69. George MS, Rush AJ, Marangell LB, et al. A one-year comparison of vagus nerve stimulation with treatment as usual for treatment-resistant depression. *Biol Psychiatry*. 2005;58(5):364–73.

70. Rush AJ, Sackeim HA, Marangell LB, et al. Effects of 12 months of vagus nerve stimulation in treatment-resistant depression: a naturalistic study. *Biol Psychiatry*. 2005;58(5):355–63.

71. Rush AJ, Marangell LB, Sackeim HA, et al. Vagus nerve stimulation for treatment-resistant depression: a randomized, controlled acute phase trial. *Biol Psychiatry*. 2005;58(5):347–54.

72. Marangell L, Suppes T, Zboyan H, et al. *Vagus Nerve Stimulation for the Treatment of Rapid Cycling Bipolar Disorder*. Poster presented at the 44th American College of Neuropsychopharmacology (ACNP) Annual Meeting, Waikoloa, Hawaii; December 11-15, 2005.

73. Fitzgerald PB, Benitez J, de Castella A, et al. A randomized, controlled trial of sequential bilateral repetitive transcranial magnetic stimulation for treatment-resistant depression. *Am J Psychiatry*. 2006;163(1):88–94.

74. Mitchell PB, Loo CK. Transcranial magnetic stimulation for depression. *Aust N Z J Psychiatry*. 2006;40:406–13.

75. Saba G, Rocamora JF, Kalalou K, et al. Repetitive transcranial magnetic stimulation as an add-on therapy in the treatment of mania: a case series of eight patients. *Psychiatry Res*. 2004;128:199–202.

76. Maihöfner C, Ropohlb A, Reulbach U, et al. Effects of repetitive transcranial magnetic stimulation in depression: a magnetoencephalographic study. *Neuroreport*. 2005;16:1839–42.

77. Kozel FA, George MS. Meta-analysis of left prefrontal repetitive transcranial magnetic stimulation (rTMS) to treat depression. *J Psychiatr Pract*. 2002;8(5):270–5.

78. Nahas Z, Kozel FA, Li X, et al. Left prefrontal transcranial magnetic stimulation (TMS) treatment of depression in bipolar affective disorder: a pilot study of acute safety and efficacy. *Bipolar Disord*. 2003;5:40–7.

INTRODUCTION

PRESENTATION

CLINICAL PROCESS

PHARMACOTHERAPY

RESOURCES

Chapter 11: Manage the Illness

Optimal bipolar treatment will always balance considerations of efficacy, tolerability and safety. A growing body of evidence suggests that:

- The depressive phase of bipolar illness could be responsible for most of the disorder's associated morbidity and mortality.[1, 2]
- Sub-syndromal illness is both impairing and predictive of future relapse into syndromal episodes.[3, 4]

As a result, every effort should be made to avoid relapse within the limits of tolerability and safety. This will usually require combinations of effective agents. Additionally, maintenance therapy must focus on issues of patient adherence to treatment plans. Despite the efficacy of acute treatment, patients are often non-adherent for a variety of reasons, not the least of which involve understanding the chronic nature of the disease, dealing with the stigmas associated with the diagnosis, and handling medication side effects. Non-adherence is associated with relapse and, perhaps, refractory status. Strategies to improve adherence and treatment outcome are not well researched at this time.

Primary care physicians may want to review the material on page 150 through 151 of chapter 10 related to:

- *Illness phase*
- *Severity*
- *Clinician readiness/ scope of practice*
- *Patient readiness*
- *Quality of the therapeutic alliance*
- *Psychosocial considerations*

It is helpful to track your responses throughout the course of a patient's treatment to determine when and if consultation with and/or referral to a specialist in treating bipolar disorder may be appropriate.

Maintenance therapy is indicated for patients with bipolar disorder after an episode of mania or depression.[5-7] Although studies are limited, it is also reasonable to institute maintenance therapy in patients with bipolar II disorder, as the overall course, severity, and functional impacts are substantial.[8]

This chapter presents:

- Goals of maintenance therapy.

- An overview of medications used for maintenance therapy, including TIMA recommendations for bipolar I disorder. See later chapters for detailed information, such as dosing and side effects (chapters 12–14) and clinical trial results (chapter 14).

- The impacts and issues surrounding treatment adherence and in balancing safety, efficacy, and tolerability in bipolar treatment.

- Maintenance treatment information for Holly and Janice, two case study patients featured throughout this clinical process section.

Maintenance Therapy Goals

One of the most important long-term goals of therapy in patients with bipolar disorder is to prevent the recurrence of additional mood episodes. Since approximately 90 percent of patients who experience a manic episode will have recurrent episodes, it is important not only to treat the initial manic/hypomanic or major depressive episode, but also to prevent subclinical or clinical relapses.[8] Maintenance therapy is intended to achieve this objective.

Maintenance therapy should also reduce the likelihood that the patient will experience sub-syndromal symptoms. Appropriate maintenance therapy should improve functional outcomes and decrease suicide risk, frequency of cycling, and mood instability.

The approach to maintenance therapy for patients with bipolar disorder also requires ongoing reevaluation of the patient, their specific "bipolarity," and the clinician's scope of practice/comfort level with involvement in ongoing treatment. This reevaluation involves many of the same considerations of initial treatment planning both for those involved in the patient's care and for the patient and the patient's family, such as:

- **Severity of disease** — At this point in the patient's treatment, has the severity of the disease changed in such a way as to require more of a collaborative care approach? What is the patient's risk for recurrence?

- **Presence of rapid cycling and/or psychosis** — If the patient is experiencing these types of breakthrough symptoms, is there a problem with either treatment resistance or medication adherence?

- **Reasonable patient preferences** — What side effects is the patient experiencing, and how tolerable are these side effects versus those caused by other treatments?

- **Co-occurring medical or psychiatric illnesses** — Are there ongoing effects of comorbid substance abuse, anxiety, or other illnesses that need to be dealt with more aggressively in order to achieve better mood stability?

Medication Treatments for Maintaining Stability

There are relatively few scientific studies on the long-term management of patients with bipolar disorder. In practice, virtually all patients will need ongoing antimanic medication to prevent symptom relapse. For those taking a combination of mood stabilizers and undergoing medication changes, the clinician should taper one medication either associated with side effects or limited partial response, while continuing other medications.

Current general practice guidelines recommend the use of lifetime treatment after two manic episodes, or after one episode if severe and/or a significant family history of bipolar or major depressive disorder exists.

See chapter 14 for detailed information on clinical trial results for medications in bipolar maintenance treatment. Chapters 12 and 13 provide in-depth information on specific antimanic and antidepressant medications, including side effects and dosing guidelines.

INTRODUCTION

PRESENTATION

CLINICAL PROCESS

PHARMACOTHERAPY

RESOURCES

Current recommendations are to gradually taper antidepressant treatment after symptom remission and after a period of stability lasting two to four months. However, some patients with bipolar disorder may need ongoing antidepressant treatment along with antimanic agents. As early as the 1970s, researchers noticed that medications necessary for minimizing manic symptoms sometimes pushed the brain below a euthymic level, thus necessitating use of antidepressants to balance the brain chemistry.

Mood stabilizer therapy is the mainstay of maintenance therapy for patients with bipolar disorder. While monotherapy would be ideal, in practice many patients require more than one medication for long-term mood stabilization.

When patients continue to experience breakthrough symptoms or mood instability, the clinician should first ensure that drug levels are within the therapeutic range. If levels are in the low- to mid-range and side effects are minimal, increase maintenance dosing to achieve a level at the higher end of the therapeutic or dose range.

In the TIMA 2005 Update to the Algorithms of Treatment for bipolar I disorder, the panel developed maintenance treatment recommendations based on the nature of the most recent episode: hypomanic/manic vs. depressed.[9] Maintenance recommendations are presented as "levels" versus specified algorithms because of the more limited body of evidence available.

These recommendations, presented in figure 11.1 on the next page, reflect results from recent placebo-controlled trials primarily for monotherapy in long-term maintenance treatment. The TIMA guidelines are ranked by level of evidence in support of maintenance use in combination with expert consensus. Importantly, longer-term studies such as

Analogous to managing heart failure in primary practice, bipolar maintenance therapy should seek to reach target doses of selected agents, as these represent the benchmarks of randomized trials from which guidelines are drawn.

these generally have low study completion rates, necessitating more research on the role of combination therapy versus monotherapy for maintenance treatment. Continuation of therapies that achieved remission of symptoms is always an optimal maintenance strategy.

Figure 11.1   TIMA Recommendations for Maintenance Treatment[9]

	BD-I Maintenance Treatment After Hypomanic, Manic or Mixed Episodes
Level 1	Lithium (Li) or valproate (VPA) if frequent, recent, or severe mania
	Lamotrigine (LTG) acceptable otherwise
	Olanzapine (OLZ) as an alternative
Level 2*	Aripiprazole (ARP)
Level 3*	Carbamazepine (CBZ)
	Clozapine (CLOZ) if treatment-resistant
Level 4*	Quetiapine (QTP), risperidone (RIS), ziprasidone (ZIP)
Level 5*	Typical antipsychotics, oxcarbazepine (OXC), electroconvulsive therapy (ECT)
	BD-I Maintenance Treatment After Depressive Episodes
Level 1	LTG + antimanic agent if recent and/or severe manic history
	LTG monotherapy acceptable otherwise
Level 2*	Li
Level 3*	Antimanic + antidepressant effective in past, including olanzapine-fluoxetine combination (OFC)
Level 4*	VPA, CBZ, atypical antipsychotics (ARP, OLZ, QTP, RIS, ZIP)
	CLOZ if treatment-resistant
Level 5*	Typical antipsychotics, OXC, ECT

*If treatments at earlier levels ineffective or not tolerated
Adapted from Suppes T, et al. (2005), *J Clin Psychiatry*, 66(7):870-86.[9]

Sidebar tabs: INTRODUCTION · PRESENTATION · CLINICAL PROCESS · PHARMACOTHERAPY · RESOURCES

Mood Stabilizers

As mood stabilizers recommended for maintenance therapy, lithium has robust evidence and valproic acid formulations also have demonstrated efficacy.[10] Lamotrigine, an antiepileptic medication, also has mood-stabilizing properties. The combination of lithium for prevention of mania and lamotrigine for depression control may be particularly valuable, although this has not yet been demonstrated in a randomized, controlled trial.

To maximize outcomes of lithium maintenance therapy, serum lithium levels usually need to be maintained at a level of 0.6–0.8 mEq/L or higher.[6] Several studies have demonstrated that lithium levels in the 0.4 mEq/L to 0.6 mEq/L range are associated with relapse rates and sub-syndromal manifestations that are 2.6-fold greater than those seen in patients with levels of 0.8 mEq/L or greater.[7, 11] Importantly, however, higher lithium levels are associated with greater toxicity and associated discontinuations. Therefore, the optimal serum lithium level in an individual patient is one that achieves the best efficacy-tolerability ratio.

When considering lithium maintenance therapy, it is important to consider factors that may reduce response to the medication (figure 11.2, below).[12]

Figure 11.2 Factors Associated with Decreased Response to Lithium Maintenance Therapy[12]

- Rapid cycling
- Multiple prior mood episodes
- Absence of a family history of mood disorders
- Associated alcohol or substance use disorder
- Episode sequence of depression-mania-euthymia

Atypical Antipsychotics (AAPs)

Atypical antipsychotics (especially clozapine, olanzapine, and aripiprazole) represent an evidence-based approach and a favorable risk-benefit profile in the long-term treatment of acute bipolar disorder relative to the older typical antipsychotics. They are particularly useful when the episode is severe or when it is accompanied by psychotic manifestations. Evolving evidence suggests that these agents (and probable others) may have a role in long-term therapy of patients with bipolar disorder.

HOLLY

Holly does well for the next six months and then returns for an unscheduled visit to report that she has felt worse for several weeks. Her psychotherapist called to alert her primary care physician to her difficulties and recommended a visit for a medication adjustment.

Holly stated that her mood had become "fragile," and she experienced sudden, intense depressions of five to six days duration when her sadness reappeared, combined at times with a sense of restlessness. Suicidal thoughts had been gone for months, but had returned as well. Following these brief depressions, she switched to a two- to three-day period of hypomania before "crashing" back into a depression. She could identify no current triggers for this. She reported that she was working well with her psychotherapist and learning a great deal. She was not acutely suicidal.

Routine blood work revealed a comprehensive metabolic panel to be within normal limits and a thyroid stimulating hormone level of 1.938 μIU/ml (normal 0.350 to 5.500μIU/ml).

Psychopharmacologic options at this time included optimizing her lamotrigine dose or adding an additional mood stabilizer. She agreed to weekly visits. Her lamotrigine dose was increased to 300 mg daily, but without benefit over the next three weeks. At that point, her lamotrigine dose was reduced to 200 mg daily. Because of the recent evidence for quetiapine in bipolar II depressed patients, quetiapine was added with evening doses beginning with 50 mg on day 1, 100 mg on day 2, 200 mg on day 3, and 300 mg on subsequent days.

*Holly experienced modest somnolence (feeling somewhat
sleepy until 11:00 the next morning), which abated after
one to two weeks, and improvement in her mood and mood
stability. Over the next four to six weeks, she regained her
remitted status and remained in remission during the next
12 months.*

Balancing Safety, Efficacy, and Tolerability

Key side effects that patients with bipolar disorder may experience with medication therapy include appetite changes
and weight gain, gastrointestinal upset, tremor, sedation,
cognitive problems (concentration, memory, difficulties
with organization and arithmetic, etc.), extrapyramidal
symptoms (Parkinson-like side effects, such as akathisia,
flat facial expression, stiff muscles, and slowed movements), tardive dyskinesia (development of involuntary
motor movements, which may persist beyond use of the
medication — usually associated with older antipsychotics), insomnia, and sexual dysfunction.

A key clinical treatment issue in managing patients'
medications is how changes are made. Always overlap a

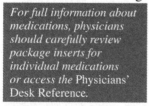
*For full information about
medications, physicians
should carefully review
package inserts for
individual medications
or access the* Physicians'
Desk Reference.

new medication with ongoing
medications, and gradually
taper any medication being
discontinued unless there is a
medical necessity to rapidly
stop (e.g., allergic reaction or
severe side effects). Figure

11.3, on pages 208 and 209, presents a general summary of
recommendations for these side effects. This list is neither
comprehensive nor intended to replace medical evaluation of
side effects, but provides a general example of many useful
approaches to side effects in this population.

Another critical aspect of managing side effects is the
monitoring for potential drug interactions. Medications
taken for heart, renal, endocrinologic, or hepatic disease
may interact with a mood stabilizer like lithium or other

antimanic/antidepressive medications. Patients should also be asked about over-the-counter medication use.

Clinicians need to carefully discuss both response and side effects with patients, emphasizing that, for most patients, bipolar disorder requires lifelong treatment.

JANICE

Lamotrigine was eventually added to Janice's treatment with olanzapine to manage her persistent depressive symptoms. Success with this approach was marked in terms of being noticeable to Janice and demonstrable on her PHQ-9 results when followed longitudinally. However, it was not a complete success: Mild to moderate depressive episodes continued for the next 18 months. Bupropion was added on two occasions for the treatment of acute depressive episodes with only modest success — less than 50 percent reduction in depression symptoms. However, racing thoughts and impulsivity (with decreased need for sleep) emerged on each occasion.

Weight was a chronic concern for Janice. She did not gain tremendous weight with olanzapine; however, she felt it hindered her ability to diet and achieve her goal weight. Eventually, because of repeated episodes of depression and weight issues, lithium was substituted for olanzapine with good success in the remission of her depression symptoms. Her weight problem was not improved; however, she experienced a robust, sustained remission over the next year of follow-up. In fact, Janice kept her job and got a promotion to a better position in the company about a year after the illness presented. Her primary relationships improved as well, and she is getting married later this year.

INTRODUCTION

PRESENTATION

CLINICAL PROCESS

PHARMACOTHERAPY

RESOURCES

Figure 11.3 Managing Medication Side Effects

GI Upset	• Administer medication with food and large quantities of liquid. • Consider lowering dose, if possible. • Use sustained-release preparations of medications, when available. • Some data suggest that this side effect can be successfully treated with H^2 blockers (e.g., cimetidine, ranitidine).
Tremor	**Enhanced physiologic tremor** — A fine tremor of approximately 8–10 Hz., made worse when hands are outstretched. • Check blood levels of medication. • Decrease dose, divide dose, or change to slow-absorption preparation of the medication. • Optionally, prescribe propranolol at 20–30 mg, 3 times daily, or at 80 mg long-acting, daily. **Parkinsonian tremor** — Coarse tremor at rest of approximately 4–6 Hz. • Decrease dose, divide dose, use bedtime dosing, or switch to alternate medication. • Choose among pharmacological treatments, including: benztropine 1–2 mg twice daily; amantadine 100 mg, 2 or 3 times daily; and diphenhydramine 25–50 mg, 2 or 3 times daily.
Sedation	• Change to bedtime dosing. • Substitute a less-sedating, alternative medication.
Sexual Dysfunction	• Add yohimbine at 4–7.5 mg, 3 times a day, • or add cyproheptadine at 4–8 mg given shortly before sexual intercourse, • or give the antidepressant bupropion at dosages of 75–300 mg per day. Bupropion has the advantage of potentially also augmenting the antidepressant efficacy of an SSRI.

Figure 11.3 (continued)

Extrapyramidal Symptoms (EPS)	**Note:** This is usually seen with older antipsychotics. • Treat tremor as suggested above. • Reduce dose of antipsychotic medication. • For akathisia, prescribe propranolol (20–30 mg, 3 times a day; or 80 mg slow-absorbing form, daily), benztropine, amantadine, or diphenhydramine. If these are ineffective, alternatives include clonidine (0.1 mg, 3 times a day) and lorazepam (1–2 mg, 2–3 times daily). • For dystonic reactions, seek prevention with benztropine 1 mg, 2 or 3 times daily for the first few days of antipsychotic therapy. Acute dystonic reactions are generally managed with benztropine 1–2 mg or lorazepam 1 mg intramuscular.
Tardive Dyskinesia (TD)	• Prescribe antipsychotics in the lowest dose necessary for the shortest time possible. • Consider alternatives for mood stabilization and control of agitation. • Use atypical antipsychotic medications, which appear to have a lower incidence of TD. • Prescribe vitamin E, as some evidence exists that vitamin E given in high doses (>1,000 units per day) may decrease some symptoms of TD for some patients.
Insomnia	• Use morning dosing, or spread total daily dose as early in the day as possible. • Use QHS dosing for any potentially sedating medications. • Use zolpidem (5–10 mg) at bedtime, zaleplon (5–20 mg; 10 mg recommended dose) at bedtime, or a benzodiazepine (such as temazepam, 15–30 mg) at night. Antipsychotics should always be considered second- or third-line agents for insomnia because of their risk of extrapyramidal symptoms and tardive dyskinesia. Avoid use of higher doses of trazodone for sleep, as it is an antidepressant and thus has the potential for destabilizing and increasing symptoms of mania in patients with bipolar disorder. Benzodiazepines are best avoided in patients with prior history of substance abuse/dependence or who are at risk for substance abuse. For these patients, nonaddicting agents are preferred.

INTRODUCTION

PRESENTATION

CLINICAL PROCESS

PHARMACOTHERAPY

RESOURCES

Facilitating Medication Adherence

Despite advances in effective medication treatments for bipolar disorder, some people's symptoms do not completely remit or disappear. As medication combinations become more complex, the likelihood of side effects (e.g., weight gain, nausea, and cognitive "dullness") increases and patients' willingness to comply with prescribed regimens decreases. Key reasons for patients to lapse in or totally stop taking their medications include:

- Not wanting to lose what many patients perceive as the more satisfying and productive symptom spectrum (e.g., hypomania), a situation that makes side effects even more intolerable

- Finding the negative side effects of some medications intolerable

- Mistakenly thinking that, by not experiencing an episode in some time, they have been "cured" and no longer require treatment

Research indicates that, in the first year of treatment, one-half to two-thirds of patients fail to comply with medication treatment. Some data suggest that most patients remain fully compliant with mood-stabilizing medication for only two months.[13–16]

In a 2005 study of cultural issues involved with treating bipolar disorder, Fleck et al. found that ethnicity plays a role in reasons for nonadherence.[17] Specifically, African-American participants were more likely to cite patient-related factors associated with nonadherence , specifically the fear of becoming addicted to medications and feeling that medications were symbols of mental illness, than were Caucasian participants. Caucasians were more likely to cite medication-related factors — efficacy, substance use, course of illness, side effects, and insight or regard for illness — as reasons for not taking their medications as prescribed.[17]

Another issue in medication adherence/compliance involves cost in terms of hospitalizations of patients who adhere to their medication regimens vs. of those who do not. Results from a 2002 study of 98 patients with mood disorders taking prescribed antimanic medications indicate that increased adherence leads to fewer symptoms and less hospitalization. In addition, 36 percent of those studied had less than optimal serum plasma levels, yet good adherence appeared to have a protective effect.[18] Other recent research measured the costs of nonadherence in irregular versus regular medication users, finding the following:[19]

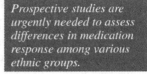

Prospective studies are urgently needed to assess differences in medication response among various ethnic groups.

- **Hospitalization rates** — 73 percent for irregular medication users vs. 31 percent for regular medication users
- **Mean length of stay** — 37 days for irregular medication users vs. 4 days for regular medication users
- **Hospitalization costs** — $9,701 for irregular medication users vs. $1,657 for regular ones

Optimum treatment of bipolar disorder occurs when psychosocial interventions augment pharmacological treatments. Several studies suggest that psychoeducation and interventions that address medication adherence substantially improve both adherence to treatment and clinical and functional outcomes. For example, Colom et al. found that those patients participating in a psychoeducation program enjoyed a longer period of stability and fewer days of hospitalization (4.75 vs. 14.83 days for the control group) over a 24-month follow-up period.[20]

Because of these issues, psychosocial interventions for bipolar disorder emphasize education on the recurrent and lifelong nature of this illness and on the importance of medication compliance.

Preventing Relapse

Bipolar disorder is a lifelong condition characterized by repeated mood episodes. Despite previously adequate treatment, individuals can experience relapse or the emergence of a new mood episode (depression, hypomania, mania, or mixed) after achieving remission.

The efficacy of lithium, lamotrigine, and olanzapine in relapse prevention in bipolar I disorder has been demonstrated in placebo-controlled, long-term trials.[21–26] Valproate, carbamazepine, clozapine, and aripiprazole also appear to have efficacy in controlled trails studying maintenance treatment of bipolar disorder.[27–33] Patients treated with a mood stabilizer plus an atypical antipsychotic also appear to have a lower risk of relapse if the combination is continued as maintenance treatment.[32, 34–39]

Depressive relapse is thought to be the most frequent problem during maintenance therapy. As with case study patient Holly, agents with efficacy for bipolar depression (e.g., quetiapine) may be reasonable interventions for acute treatment, where continuation treatment decisions are guided by periodic assessment. Information on agents with efficacy in both acute and maintenance phases is the focus of current research. Clinical judgement should be used in the absence of controlled data.

Psychosocial treatment may augment the effects of pharmacotherapy in preventing relapse by teaching patients and their loved ones to identify early warning signs that might signal an imminent episode. In general, as patients experience longer intervals of wellness, their risk of a new episode decreases.[40]

Patients need to learn to recognize external events that may trigger an increase in symptoms (e.g., an upcoming family event that has been stressful in the past). Additionally, psychosocial treatment can help individuals learn to monitor themselves for unique behaviors that are reliable warning signs of an increase in symptoms or an emergent episode. Warning signs (e.g., restless sleep, insomnia, increased irritability, or more frequent purchase of lottery tickets) tend to be very unique for each individual, but can be identified, monitored, and acted upon as a helpful relapse prevention tool. Along with recognition of the early warning signs, patients should have a plan for dealing with them, including concrete actions one can quickly take to stabilize the situation, such as calling the clinician.

References for Chapter 11

1. Manning JS. Burden of illness in bipolar depression. *Prim Care Companion J Clin Psychiatry*. 2005;7(6):259–67.

2. Post RM Denicoff KD, Leverich GS, et al. Morbidity in 258 bipolar outpatients followed for 1 year with daily prospective ratings on the NIMH life chart method. *J Clin Psychiatry*. 2003;64(6):680–90; quiz 738–9.

3. Perlis RH Ostacher MJ, Patel JK, et al. Predictors of recurrence in bipolar disorder: primary outcomes from the Systematic Treatment Enhancement Program for Bipolar Disorder (STEP-BD). *Am J Psychiatry*. 2006Feb;163(2):217–24.

4. Altshuler LL, Post RM, Black DO, et al. Subsyndromal depressive symptoms are associated with functional impairment in patients with bipolar disorder. *J Clin Psychiatry*. 2006; In press.

5. Keck PE Jr, Welge JA, Strakowski SM, et al. Placebo effect in randomized, controlled maintenance studies of patients with bipolar disorder. *Biol Psychiatry*. 2000;47(8):756–61.

6. Baldessarini RJ, Tondo L, Hennen J, Viguera AC. Is lithium still worth using? An update of selected recent research. *Harv Rev Psychiatry*. 2002; 10(2):59–75.

7. Keller MB, Lavori PW, Kane JM, et al. Subsyndromal symptoms in bipolar disorder. A comparison of standard and low serum levels of lithium. *Arch Gen Psychiatry*. 1992; 49(5):371–6.

8. Hopkins HS, Gelenberg AJ. Treatment of bipolar disorder: how far have we come? *Psychopharmacol Bull*. 1994;30(1):27–38.

9. Suppes T, Dennehy EB, Hirschfeld RMA, et al. The Texas Implementation of Medication Algorithms: update to the algorithms for treatment of bipolar I disorder. *J Clin Psychiatry*. 2005;66(7):870–86.

10. Keck PE, Jr, McElroy SL: Treatment of bipolar disorder. *American Psychiatric Association Textbook of Psychopharmocology*. 3rd ed. Washington, DC:APPI;2004.

11. Gelenberg AJ, Kane JM, Keller MB, et al. Comparison of standard and low serum levels of lithium for maintenance treatment of bipolar disorder. *N Engl J Med.* 1989;321(22):1489–93.

12. Bowden CL. Predictors of response to divalproex and lithium. *J Clin Psychiatr.* 1995;56(Suppl):25–30.

13. Keck PE Jr, McElroy SL, Strakowski SM, et al. Factors associated with pharmacologic noncompliance in patients with mania. *J Clin Psychiatry.* 1996;57:292–7.

14. Keck PE Jr, McElroy SL, Strakowski SM, et al. Twelve-month outcome of patients with bipolar disorder following hospitalization for a manic or mixed episode. *Am J Psychiatry.* 1998;155:646–52.

15. Johnson RE, McFarland BH. Lithium use and discontinuation in a health maintenance organization. *Am J Psychiatry.* 1996;153:993–1000.

16. Lingam R, Scott J. Treatment non-adherence in affective disorders. *Acta Psychiatr Scand.* 2002;105(3):164–72.

17. Fleck DE, Keck PE Jr, Corey KB, Strakowski SM. Factors associated with medication adherence in African American and white patients with bipolar disorder. *J Clin Psychiatry.* 2005;66(5):646–52.

18. Scott J, Pope M. Non-adherence with mood stabilizers: prevalence and predictors. *Am J Psychiatry.* 2002;159(11):1927–29.

19. Svarstad BL, Shireman TI, Sweeney JK. Using drug claims data to assess the relationship of medication adherence with hospitalization and costs. *Psychiatr Serv.* 2001;52(6):805–11.

20. Colom F, Vieta E, Martinez-Aran A, et al. A randomized trial on the efficacy of group psychoeducation in the prophylaxis of recurrences in bipolar patients whose disease is in remission. *Arch Gen Psychiatry.* 2003;60(4):402–7.

21. Keck PE Jr., Welge JA, Strakowski SM, et al. Placebo effect in random-ized, controlled maintenance studies of patients with bipolar disorder. *Biol Psychiatry.* 2000; 47(8):756–61.

22. Bowden CL, Calabrese JR, Sachs G, et al. A placebo-controlled 18-month trial of lamotrigine and lithium maintenance treatment in recently manic or hypomanic patients with bipolar I disorder. *Arch Gen Psychiatry.* 2003;60(4):392–400.

23. Calabrese JR, Bowden CL, Sachs G, et al. A placebo-controlled 18-month trial of lamotrigine and lithium maintenance treatment in recently depressed patients with bipolar I disorder. *J Clin Psychiatry.* 2003;64(9):1013–24.

24. Tohen M, Marneros A, Bowden C, et.al. Olanzapine versus lithium in relapse prevention in bipolar disorder: a randomized double-blind con-trolled 12-week trial. In *Abstracts of the New Clinical Drug Evaluation Unit Annual Meeting.* Boca Raton, FL, May 26-28, 2003.

25. Tohen M, Ketter TA, Zarate CA, et al. Olanzapine versus divalproex sodium for the treatment of acute mania and maintenance of remission: a 47-week study. *Am J Psychiatry.* 2003;160(7):1263–71.

26. Tohen B, Bowden C, Calabrese J, et al. Olanzapine's efficacy for relapse prevention in bipolar disorder: a placebo-controlled, randomized, double-blind controlled 12-month trial. In *Abstracts of the Fifth International Conference on Bipolar Disorder.* Pittsburgh, PA, June 16, 2003.

27. Bowden CL, Calabrese JR, McElroy SL, et al. A randomized, placebo-controlled 12-month trial of divalproex and lithium in treatment of outpatients with bipolar I disorder. Divalproex Maintenance Study Group. *Arch Gen Psychiatry.* 2000; 57(5):481–9.

28. Revicki D, Hirschfeld R, Keck PE Jr. Cost-effectiveness of divalproex sodium vs. lithium in long-term therapy for bipolar disorder. In *American College of Neuropsychopharmacology Annual Meeting.* San Juan, PR. 1999.

29. Lambert P, Vernaud G. Comparative study of valpromide versus lithium as prophylactic treatment of affective disorders. *Nervure J Psychiatrie.* 1982;4:1–9.

30. Denicoff KD, Smith-Jackson EE, Disney ER, et al. Comparative prophylactic efficacy of lithium, carbamazepine, and the combination in bipolar disorder. *J Clin Psychiatry.* 1997;58(11):470–8.

31. Greil W, Ludwig-Mayerhofer W, Erazo N, et al. Lithium versus carbamazepine in the maintenance treatment of bipolar disorders — a randomised study. *J Affect Disord.* 1997;43(2):151–61.

32. Suppes T, Webb A, Paul B, et al. Clinical outcome in a randomized 1-year trial of clozapine versus treatment as usual for patients with treatment-resistant illness and a history of mania. *Am J Psychiatry.* 1999;156(8):1164–9.

33. Keck PE Jr, Sanchez R, Marcus RN, et al. Aripiprazole for relapse prevention in bipolar disorder in a 26-week trial. Presented at *The 157th Meeting of the American Psychiatric Association,* New York, NY; May 1-6, 2004.

34. Tohen M, Chengappa KNR, Suppes T, et al. Relapse prevention in bipolar I disorder: 18-month comparison of olanzapine plus mood stabiliser v. mood stabiliser alone. *British Journal of Psychiatry.* 2004;184:337–45.

35. Vieta E, Goikolea JM, Corbella B, et al. Risperidone safety and efficacy in the treatment of bipolar and schizoaffective disorders: results from a 6-month, multicenter, open study. *J Clin Psychiatry.* 2001;62(10):818–25.

36. Vieta E, Reinares M, Corbella B, et al. Olanzapine as long-term adjunctive therapy in treatment-resistant bipolar disorder. *J Clin Psychopharacol.* 2001;21:469–73.

37. Tohen M, Chengappa KNR, Suppes T, et al. Efficacy of olanzapine in combination with valproate or lithium in the treatment of mania in patients partially nonresponsive to valproate or lithium monotherapy. *Arch Gen Psychiatry.* 2002;59:62–9.

INTRODUCTION

PRESENTATION

CLINICAL PROCESS

PHARMACOTHERAPY

RESOURCES

38. Hardoy MC, Garofalo A, Carpiniello B, et al. Combination quetiapine therapy in the long-term treatment of patients with bipolar I disorder. *Clin Pract Epidemol Ment Health.* 2005;1:7.

39. Pae CU, Kim TS, Kim JJ, et al. Long-term treatment of adjunctive quetiapine for bipolar mania. *Prog in Neuropsychopharmacol.* 2005;29:763–6.

40. Tohen M, Waternaux CM, Tsuang MT. Outcome in mania: A 4-year prospective follow-up of 75 patients utilizing survival analysis. *Arch Gen Psychiatry.* 1990;47:1106–11.

Chapter 12: Antimanic Medications

Antimanic agents are used to treat patients with bipolar disorder experiencing either manic or mixed episodes. This chapter discusses medications found to be effective in the treatment of acute mania and mixed episodes in patients with bipolar I disorder. There are four types of medications used for antimanic therapy listed below (those in bold type have been specifically approved by the FDA for the treatment of **acute bipolar mania**):

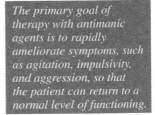

The primary goal of therapy with antimanic agents is to rapidly ameliorate symptoms, such as agitation, impulsivity, and aggression, so that the patient can return to a normal level of functioning.

- **Lithium**, which has been the mainstay of treatment for acute mania since approved in 1970.

- Some antiepileptic drugs (AEDs), including **divalproex sodium** and **carbamazepine ER**, which have been studied the most extensively for their use in antimanic therapy.

- Typical antipsychotics (e.g., **chlorpromazine**, haloperidol, perphenazine, and thioridazine) have antimanic efficacy, particularly in patients with significant agitation. Because of neurological and neuroendocrinological side effects, these medications have been largely supplanted by the atypical antipsychotics.

- Atypical antipsychotics (sometimes referred to as newer- or second-generation psychotropics) include **olanzapine**, clozapine, **risperidone**, **quetiapine**, **ziprasidone**, and **aripiprazole**. These agents share many pharmacodynamic/pharmacokinetic properties, but have different adverse effects.

SECTION D: BIPOLAR DISORDER PHARMACOTHERAPY

Figure 12.1, below, provides dosing information for the most commonly prescribed antimanic agents.

Figure 12.1   Overview of Antimanic Agent Dosing

	Antimanic Agent	Dose Range*	Admin. Schedule
	Lithium	0.6/1.0–1.2 mEq/L	BID or QHS
Anticonvulsants	Divalproex, valproate, valproic acid	80–125 µg/mL (acute) 50–125 µg/mL (overall)	BID or QHS
	Carbamazepine ER	400–1600 units (4–12 µg/mL)	BID or QD
	Oxcarbazepine	600–2400	BID or TID
Atypical Antipsychotics**	Clozapine	75–900	QHS
	Olanzapine	10–20	QHS
	Quetiapine	400–800	BID
	Risperidone	2–6	BID or QHS
	Ziprasidone	120–160	BID
	Aripiprazole	10–30	QHS

*Doses used for maintenance therapy may be lower.

** Also referred to as "Newer Generation Psychotropics"

Figure 12.2 (on pages 219 and 220) provides a brief overview of information on side effects and other concerns covered in detail throughout this chapter.

Figure 12.2 Overview of Antimanic Agent Side Effects and Special Concerns

Antimanic Agent	Side Effects*	Concerns
Lithium	Tremor, drowsiness, nausea/vomiting, increased urine output, muscle weakness, thirst, dry mouth, cognitive impairment	Toxicity risk increases at levels above 1.5 mEq/L. Above 2.0 mEq/L, life-threatening side effects may occur.
Anticonvulsants		
Divalproex, valproate, valproic acid (Divalproex sodium, the enteric-coated form of valproate, is the FDA-approved form for treatment of acute mania.)	Nausea/vomiting, increased appetite with weight gain, sedation, hair loss, reversible increases in liver function tests, reversible thrombocytopenia, and rarely pancreatitis and liver failure	Valproate can increase free warfarin levels and increase bleeding time. Use of both medications should be monitored carefully. Aspirin inhibits valproate metabolism.
Carbamazepine ER	Dizziness, drowsiness, double vision, fatigue, nausea, vomiting, ataxia, tremor, discomfort due to indigestion, abnormal gait, hyponatremia, rash; rare Stevens-Johnson syndrome; agranulocytosis	For non-ER formulation, high serum levels may be indicative of side effect risk
Oxcarbazepine	Dizziness, hyponatremia, ataxia, diplopia, headache, sedation, impaired speech, double vision, nausea and gastrointestinal upset, and reversible mild, below-normal white blood cell range. May lower oral contraceptive efficacy.	

(continued)

INTRODUCTION

PRESENTATION

CLINICAL PROCESS

PHARMACOTHERAPY

RESOURCES

Figure 12.2 (continued)

Antimanic Agent	Side Effects*	Concerns
Atypical Antipsychotics (AAPs)		
Clozapine	Sedation, weight gain,** dry mouth, constipation, and potential mental confusion, postural hypotension, rapid heart rate, excessive salivation, constipation, nausea, and vomiting	Associated incidence of agranulocytosis; lowering of seizure threshold; May lower oral contraceptive efficacy
Olanzapine	Sedation, weight gain,** dry mouth, constipation, potential mental confusion, and mild Parkinson-like symptoms (e.g., flat facial expression, stiff muscles, slowed movements)	
Quetiapine	Somnolence, dry mouth, dizziness, constipation, asthenia, abdominal pain, postural hypotension, pharyngitis, SGPT increase, dyspepsia, and weight gain**	
Risperidone	Sedation, Parkinson-like symptoms (e.g., flat facial expression, stiff muscles, slowed movements), weight gain,** hypotension, and prolactin elevation	
Ziprasidone	Sedation, QTc prolongation, nausea, vomiting, constipation, and Parkinson-like symptoms (e.g., flat facial expression, stiff muscles, slowed movements), dizziness	Should be taken with food.
Aripiprazole	Sedation, Parkinson-like symptoms (e.g., flat facial expression, stiff muscles, slowed movements), and internal feeling of restlessness or agitation (akathisia)	

*Side effects may be lower with long-acting forms of medications.

**Severity of weight gain generally rated:
  clozapine = olanzapine > quetiapine = risperidone > aripiprazole = ziprasidone.

Lithium

Lithium (Li⁺) is a monovalent cation that shares some of the properties of other cations, such as sodium (Na⁺) and potassium (K⁺). Although trace amounts are present in animal tissues, the cation has no known physiological role.

Clinical Trial Results

Lithium has been shown to be superior to placebo for the treatment of acute mania.[1] Lithium appears to be most effective in patients with elated or classical manic symptoms who lack a history of frequent mood episodes. It also appears to be less effective in patients with mixed (dysphoric) episodes or rapid cycling.[2]

Pharmacology

Although a number of cellular effects of lithium have been discovered, the precise mechanism behind the medication's mood-stabilizing properties is unknown. Possible explanations include its effects upon protein kinases, G proteins, and/or inhibition of inositol monophosphatase.

Lithium is readily absorbed from the gastrointestinal tract; almost all administered medication enters the plasma within eight hours. After an oral dose, peak plasma levels appear within two to four hours.[3] Since it is a small hydrophilic molecule, lithium's volume of distribution is approximately that of total body water. However, this volume is significantly less than that of other psychotropic medications that are both lipophilic and protein bound. Lithium passes slowly through the blood-brain barrier, and has final concentrations within the cerebrospinal fluid of 40 to 50 percent.

The medication is excreted almost completely by the kidneys; approximately one to two thirds are excreted within 12 hours of administration. After glomerular filtration, approximately 80 percent of lithium is reabsorbed by the proximal convoluted tubules (PCT). Since it shares reabsorption with sodium, renal mechanisms will increase PCT lithium absorption in patients with decreased concentrations of sodium in the glomerular filtrate. Since plasma lithium is a function of the dose administered and the patient's renal function, plasma levels of the medication will remain remarkably constant in a given individual.

Lithium Side Effects/Drug Interactions

Figure 12.3, on the next two pages, provides detailed information on management of common lithium side effects.

Many medications can alter serum lithium levels:

- During the initial phases of therapy
- When the patient has a medical illness
- When the patient is treated with any new medication that can alter lithium excretion

In patients treated with lithium and an antipsychotic, the antiemetic activity of the antipsychotic can mask some of the gastrointestinal symptoms of lithium toxicity. Therefore, it is imperative that patients have their serum lithium levels monitored regularly. (See figure 12.4, on page 224, and the *Physicians' Desk Reference* for a comprehensive list of medications affecting serum lithium levels.)

Figure 12.3 Management of Side Effects Associated with Lithium

Side Effects/Comments	Treatment Considerations
Postabsorptive syndrome — GI discomfort, nausea, weakness, vertigo due to a rapid rise in plasma lithium levels; subsides over time	• Give all at bedtime. • Try alternative preparations.
Fine tremors of the hands; fatigue can be common and persistent	• Check serum level. • Use propranolol or similar medication.
Thirst, polydipsia, polyuria, low urine specific gravity • Drug-induced abnormalities occur in renal function because of decreased renal response to antidiuretic hormone. • Some patients may continue to have impaired ability to concentrate. • Nephrogenic diabetes insipidus may occur.	• Polyuria can sometimes be managed by administering the medication once daily at bedtime. • May need dose reduction as well as adequate fluid and electrolyte replacement. • Thiazide may be required for severe symptoms, but electrolytes should be monitored, potassium supplementation may be needed, and lithium dose should be reduced. • Potassium-sparing diuretics (e.g., amiloride) can be effective and will usually not increase potassium excretion or lithium reabsorption.
Interstitial fibrosis, glomerular sclerosis, impaired water reabsorption, increased serum creatinine • Associated with long-term lithium use in some instances	• Monitor kidney function initially and then biannually.
Repolarization abnormalities on electrocardiogram (ECG) — conduction block or arrhythmia in some instances	• ECG usually indicated prior to initiating treatment in an individual over age 40.

(continued)

Figure 12.3   (continued)

Side Effects/Comments	Treatment Considerations
Hypothyroidism • More common in women • Affects up to one third of patients treated with lithium • May appear after the patient has been treated for 6 to 18 months • May be accompanied by rapid cycling • Associated risk of depression for patients who develop lithium-induced hypothyroidism	• Levothyroxine can be used while the patient is maintained on lithium. • Thyroid hormone replacement therapy and substitution of another mood stabilizer can be considered if rapid cycling or depression occur. • Check thyroid stimulating hormone level 1-2 times/year.
Dermatologic changes — pustular acne, exacerbation or precipitation of psoriasis, inhibition of anti-psoriatic therapy[4]	• Treat empirically.

Figure 12.4   Drugs that Affect Serum Lithium Levels

Increased Effect	Decreased Effect
Thiazide	Acetazolamide
Furosemide	Sodium bicarbonate
Spironolactone	Sodium chloride
Methyldopa	Theophylline
Indomethacin	Mannitol
Phenylbutazone	
Piroxicam	
Ibuprofen	

Administration

Primary Considerations

Before treatment begins, the patient's history and physical examination should be reviewed to address any issues in organ systems likely to be affected by the medication (e.g., endocrine, cardiovascular, genitourinary, skin). The patient should also be educated about lithium's potential toxicities. For obvious reasons, laboratory studies should include baseline electrolytes, chemistry, urinalysis, renal function, pregnancy, thyroid-stimulating hormone, and electrocardiogram (when appropriate).

Dosage Selection

Selection of the total daily dose should be based on age, weight, and other medical considerations. To minimize side effects, the total lithium dose is usually administered in three divided doses or at bedtime (QHS). The dose is usually kept low (e.g., 300-600 mg/d) and then titrated upward to the therapeutic target of 0.5 to 1.2 mEq/L. This usually requires 900 to 1800 mg/d (15 to 20 mg/kg).

In an attempt to balance side effects with therapeutic activity, lithium levels in the middle to upper range (0.8 to 1.2 mEq/L) are often required for the treatment of acute mania.

Titration

The rate of titration appears to affect the rapidity of response to lithium and other mood stabilizers.[1] While randomized clinical trials document symptomatic improvement within seven to 14 days, a pilot study demonstrated that patients whose dose levels were rapidly titrated to therapeutic concentrations within 24 hours experienced a significant reduction in symptoms within a span of five days.[4]

Long-Term Management

During the first six months of therapy, lithium levels should be monitored regularly, and renal and thyroid function also should be assessed. In a stable and responsible patient, testing can then be reduced to biannually unless breakthrough occurs, toxic manifestations develop, a general medical condition intervenes, or the patient's medication changes.[5]

Toxicity

Lithium toxicity is related to serum drug levels and is most common with serum lithium levels of 1.5 mEq/L or greater.[5] Potentially life-threatening side effects are common when drug levels exceed 2.0 mEq/L. At lower levels, manifestations of toxicity are those described under adverse events.

*The risk of adverse effects with lithium is a function of **both** a high serum level **and** the duration of exposure to a high level.*

At higher concentrations, however, symptoms increase in severity and may be accompanied by neurologic impairments, seizures, coma, and cardiac arrhythmias.

Anticonvulsants

Anticonvulsants found to have mood-stabilizing properties include valproate, carbamazepine, and lamotrigine (in maintenance use — see chapter 14).

Potential mechanisms of action of anticonvulsants in bipolar disorder include:

- Altering sodium and potassium fluxes via ion channels
- Upregulation of inhibitory and downregulation of excitatory neurotransmitters
- Downregulation of excitatory neurotransmitters
- Modulation of second messenger systems

Divalproex/Valproate/Valproic Acid

Valproic acid is a simple, branched-chain carboxylic acid. Its anticonvulsant properties were discovered when it was used as a vehicle for medications being screened for antiepileptic activity.

Clinical Trial Results

Divalproex sodium (the enteric-coated form of valproic acid) is FDA-indicated for the treatment of the manic episodes associated with bipolar disorder. Valproic acid and related formulations have superior efficacy compared with placebo and comparable activity with lithium, haloperidol, and olanzapine.[1] Factors associated with improved valproate versus lithium response include mixed episodes and a history of multiple prior mood episodes. The effect of valproate in comparison trials of antipsychotic compounds suggests that, like all antimanic agents, valproate has antipsychotic in addition to antimanic activity.

Pharmacology

The basis for valproate's mood stabilizing properties is not fully understood. However, since it blocks ion channels, it is thought that valproate may possibly upregulate the activity of GABAergic and downregulate the activity of glutamatergic neurotransmitters.[3]

After oral administration, valproate is rapidly absorbed, and peak serum levels are achieved within one to four hours. Once it enters the bloodstream, the medication is rapidly distributed throughout the body and is extensively protein-bound. Its half-life is typically in the 6- to 16-hour range, but half-life can be significantly altered by medications that interfere with the activities of hepatic cytochromes (such as CYP2C9) or by the process of conjugation to glucuronic acid. Once conjugated with glucuronic acid, valproate and its metabolites are predominantly excreted through the urine. Since one valproate metabolite is eliminated in the urine, its presence may register as a ketone and lead to a false positive of urinary ketones.

Side Effects/Drug Interactions

Figure 12.5, on the next page, summarizes valproate side-effect management.

Valproate can interact with a number of medications. Since the medication is largely protein-bound, it can displace other medications from serum proteins (e.g., aspirin and warfarin). Since valproate can impair nonrenal clearance of barbiturates, barbiturate drug levels should be obtained for patients receiving both drugs, and patients should be monitored for signs of neurological toxicity. Valproate inhibits the metabolism of lamotrigine; consequently, the lamotrigine dose in patients concurrently treated with valproate must be started at a dose one-half that of the recommended initial dose.

INTRODUCTION

PRESENTATION

CLINICAL PROCESS

PHARMACOTHERAPY

RESOURCES

Figure 12.5　Management of Side Effects Associated with Valproate

Side Effects/ Comments	Treatment Considerations
Sedation and GI distress common at start of treatment; symptoms usually resolve over time	• Manage persistent, drug-associated GI distress by dose-reduction, switch to another member of the valproate family (e.g., divalproex sodium for sodium valproate), and/or administer an H_2-receptor blocker (e.g., cimetidine).
Hair loss, weight gain, increased appetite	• Recommend diet and exercise. • Consider agents associated with weight loss (e.g., topiramate, zonisamide).
Mild leucopenia, thrombocytopenia, impaired platelet function	• Conduct baseline complete blood count. • Determine platelet counts and bleeding time before elective surgery and if patient has excessive bruising or hemorrhage.
Tremors may occur	• Treat with a β-blocker (e.g., propranolol).
May increase incidence of polycystic ovarian syndrome Rate of development lower than initially reported[6-9]	• Treat with oral contraceptives. • Consider potential increased sensitivity among adolescent women to hypothalmic-pituitary-adrenal (HPA) axis disruption.
Abnormal liver function; hyperammonemia in severe cases occurs in some patients	• Monitor liver function tests monthly at treatment outset, then biannually.
Hepatocellular necrosis, hemorrhagic pancreatitis, and agranulocytosis Rare idiosyncratic reactions	• Patients should be advised to seek medical help if they develop abdominal pain, jaundice, acute pharyngitis with fever, bleeding or purpura.

Administration

Preliminary considerations — Before treatment begins, the patient should undergo a comprehensive medical examination to detect evidence of preexisting hepatic or hematologic abnormalities. Baseline liver function tests and complete blood count should also be obtained.

Dosage selection — Valproate has a comparatively wide therapeutic index compared with lithium.[1] Acute antimanic activity is in the range of 50 to 125 mg/L, with improved response rates at the upper end of the therapeutic range. While some patients may require medication levels in excess of 125 mg/L to control their symptoms, side effects progressively increase above this level. Data from clinical trials indicate that divalproex therapy can be initiated safely at a dose of 20 to 30 mg/kg/d in hospitalized patients.[5] To minimize gastrointestinal and neurological toxicities, valproate treatment of outpatients is usually started at a dose of 250 mg three times a day or QHS (total dose = 750 mg/d).

Titration — Depending on the clinical response and side effects, the initial dose can be titrated upward every few days until medication levels are in the therapeutic range. However, the maximal daily adult dose should not exceed 60 mg/kg/d. Since many patients do well with once- or twice-daily dosing, the treatment regimen can be simplified when the patient stabilizes.

An extended release formulation of divalproex is now available that allows for once-daily dosing and apparently reduces the incidence of side effects. However, since the bioavailability of the extended release formulation is only approximately 85 percent of the immediate-release formulation, some patients must be treated with slightly higher doses.

INTRODUCTION

PRESENTATION

CLINICAL PROCESS

PHARMACOTHERAPY

RESOURCES

Carbamazepine

> Oxcarbazepine *is a prodrug. It is a less potent inducer of hepatic enzymes; consequently, it increases plasma levels of valproate. Additionally, unlike carbamazepine, where the metabolite is responsible for toxicity and side effects, oxcarbazepine metabolites are generally nontoxic. However, while structurally similar, it is pharmacologically a different drug and direct tests of its efficacy in bipolar disorder are needed.*

Carbamazepine is chemically related to the tricyclic antidepressants. Although initially approved for the treatment of seizures, it has also been used to treat patients with various pain syndromes, such as trigeminal neuralgia. The extended-release formulation has been approved by the FDA for treating bipolar acute manic and mixed episodes. Carbamazepine has been shown to have antimanic activity in some patients who are refractory to lithium.

Clinical Trial Results

Although superior to placebo in the treatment of acute mania, carbamazepine is often considered a second-line antimanic agent, principally because, until recently, there were few well-designed, randomized controlled trials of its use in mania.[1] Several trials have shown its efficacy to be comparable to that of lithium. Recent research focusing on the prophylactic use of carbamazepine versus lithium has had mixed results. One, two-year, randomized, double-blind study of 94 patients (not taking concurrent antipsychotics or antidepressants) found lithium superior for those patients not previously treated for mood disorders.[10] However, researchers in an earlier clinical trial cautioned that the relative efficacy of lithium over carbamazepine may be related to whether or not study participants' cases have been diagnosed with "classic" bipolar I disorder (i.e., illness lacking mood-incongruent features or comorbid psychiatric illness). Those "classic" cases appeared to do better with lithium.[11]

Pharmacology

Carbamazepine's antiepileptic activity is similar to that of phenytoin.[3] Once administered, it inhibits repolarization by downregulating the recovery rate of voltage-activated sodium channels.

Carbamazepine is slowly absorbed from the gastrointestinal tract and has peak levels four to 24 hours after a single dose. Once it enters the plasma, the majority of the medication is bound to serum proteins; approximately 20 to 30 percent of carbamazepine circulates in its free form and rapidly equilibrates in tissues other than a small, increased rate of hyponatremia. The medication is metabolized in the liver, conjugated with glucuronic acid, and excreted into the urine. Its elimination half-life is approximately 36 hours. With regular administration, however, carbamazepine upregulates the activity of hepatic enzymes, with a resultant decrease in the half-life to 16 to 24 hours.

Side Effects/Drug Interactions

Figure 12.6, on the following page, provides detailed information on common carbamazepine side effects.

Medications that increase activity of hepatic cytochromes CYP3A4, such as valproate, increase carbamazepine metabolism and lower its serum carbamazepine levels.[3] Like its tricyclic relatives, carbamazepine has anticholinergic activity that can lead to adverse events; dryness of the mouth, constipation, diplopia, blurred vision, etc.

Carbamazepine reduces plasma concentrations and efficacy of the typical antipsychotic, haloperidol. Fluoxetine, some antibiotics, and calcium channel blockers inhibit carbamazepine metabolism.

Administration

Preliminary Considerations — Before treatment begins, patients require a thorough medical history and examination to rule out preexisting disorders, including liver and blood diseases. Laboratory studies should include liver function tests, a complete blood count, and electrolytes.

INTRODUCTION

PRESENTATION

CLINICAL PROCESS

PHARMACOTHERAPY

RESOURCES

Figure 12.6   Side Effects Associated with Carbamazepine

Side Effects	Comments
CNS — drowsiness, headache	Most common
GI tract — nausea and vomiting	Dose and/or level to be checked; once-daily dosing considered
Dermatological	Non-medically serious rash; potentially fatal Stevens-Johnson syndrome and toxic epidermal necrolysis reported (rare)
Hematologic, hepatic, cardiovascular, and cutaneous reactions	Most serious
Leukopenia	Mild, transient leukopenia in approximately 10% of patients; persistent leukopenia in approximately 2% requiring medication discontinuation[1]
Fatal aplastic anemia	Approximately 1/200,000 patients
Transient elevation of hepatic enzymes	Approximately 5–10% of patients
Cardiac conduction abnormalities — bradycardia, arrhythmias, or complete heart block	Baseline ECG in patients age 45 or older

Dosage Selection — There is an inconstant relationship between the dose of carbamazepine, serum concentration, response, and side effects. Therefore, in adults, treatment is usually started at a total daily dose of 200–600 mg, divided into three or four doses.[5] While the dose can be increased in hospitalized patients in increments of 200 mg/d up to 800–1000 mg/d, slower dosage adjustments are usually indicated for less severely ill outpatients. Target serum concentrations for those with bipolar disorder have not been established; therefore, most clinicians try to maintain serum carbamazepine levels in the 4–12 μg/mL range. Since side effects are primarily due to the metabolite of carbamazepine, in some patients this can occur at low serum levels and, in others, at much higher serum levels. During the first two months of therapy, hematologic parameters and liver function tests should be monitored frequently.

> *When using the ER formulation of this medication, it is unnecessary to check serum levels.*

Other Anticonvulsants

A number of other anticonvulsants have been studied as potential antimanic agents. These include gabapentin, lamotrigine, topiramate, zonisamide, levetiracetam, tiagabine, and acamprosate. Studies of these medications have been limited by sample size and methodologic issues. However, placebo-controlled studies with lamotrigine and topiramate in acute bipolar mania were negative.[1]

Typical Antipsychotics

Typical antipsychotics include haloperidol, chlorpromazine, thioridazine, and perphenazine. These medications have antimanic efficacy, particularly in patients with significant agitation relative to lithium.[12] However, their side effects limit their long-term use. These side effects include increased risk of depression, prolactin elevation, and extrapyramidal manifestations, such as dystonias, akathisia, and tardive dyskinesia in patients with bipolar disorder. Therefore, typical antipsychotics have been largely supplanted by the atypical antipsychotics.

Atypical Antipsychotics
(Newer Generation Psychotropics)

Atypical antipsychotic agents (AAPs) are the newest additions to the psychotropic class and are remarkable for their overall improved side-effect profile. However, patients treated with antipsychotics are still at risk for extrapyramidal side effects: akathisia, tardive dyskinesia, and neuroleptic malignant syndrome. The degree of this risk has not yet been fully defined and may vary across the agents in this class.

INTRODUCTION

PRESENTATION

CLINICAL PROCESS

PHARMACOTHERAPY

RESOURCES

Characteristics of these newer generation psychotropics are:

- Minimal-to-no extrapyramidal side effects
- Intrinsic antimanic properties
- Different receptor affinities
  - D_1, D_3, D_4 >D_2; and
  - 5-HT$_{2A}$ >D_2
- Less likelihood for the neuroleptic malignant syndrome
- Greater efficacy than typical agents in some types of schizophrenia (e.g., schizophrenic deficit symptoms)
- Beneficial effects in the treatment of depressive symptoms (shown for some atypical antipsychotics)

Overall Side Effects

AAPs have varying side effect profiles related to weight gain (see pages 172 through 176 in chapter 10), glucose intolerance, hyperprolactinemia, QTc prolongation concerns, somnolence, orthostatic hypotension, and extrapyramidal symptoms (see figure 12.7 on the next page).

General Treatment Recommendations

- Prior to administration, educate patients about the identification and significance of side effects.
- Obtain baseline glucose and lipid profiles when therapy is started and then monitor at least annually. (See page 175 for ADA-recommended monitoring schedule.)
- Treat the triad of weight gain, glucose intolerance, and dyslipidemia the same as for patients with metabolic syndrome.
- Advise patients to lose weight and increase physical activity.

Figure 12.7 Comparative Side Effect Profile of Atypical Antipsychotics[13-20]

Side Effects*	Atypical Antipsychotics					
	Clozapine	Olanzapine	Risperidone	Quetiapine	Ziprasidone	Aripiprazole
Weight Gain**	3+	3+	2+	2+	+	+
Hyperprolactinemia	±	±	3+	±	±	−
Somnolence	3+	2+	+	2+	+	+
QTc Prolongation	2+	±	±	±	+	±
Orthostatic Hypotension	3+	+	2+	2+	2+	+
Extrapyramidal Symptoms	±	±	2+	±	+	+

3+ = high incidence
2+ = moderate incidence
± = equivocal findings
− = insignificant incidence

*Side effects appear to be somewhat dose related.

**Also associated with dyslipidemia.

- Address other cardiovascular risk factors, such as increased LDL-C, low HDL-C, hypertension, and cigarette-smoking.
- Analyze the risks and benefits of switching to another medication in a patient whose psychiatric disorder is well controlled.

Other clinical considerations and specific treatment recommendations for the common side effects of atypical antipsychotics are listed in Figure 12.8 Management of Side Effects of Atypical Antipsychotics, on pages 237 through 238. For each category of side effect, the following paragraphs provide a general overview.

INTRODUCTION

PRESENTATION

CLINICAL PROCESS

PHARMACOTHERAPY

RESOURCES

Weight gain — This complication is the result of medication-induced alterations in neurotransmitter circuitry involved in feeding behavior and satiety. The strongest correlation is the affinity of the drug for H_1 and possibly for $5\text{-}HT_{2C}$ receptors. The actions of the former may be due to a blockade of satiety signals from the gut, while the latter appears to act by stimulating food intake. Another possible mechanism is interference with leptin-mediated feeding behavior and total body mass of adipose tissue.

Glucose intolerance — This effect is probably multifactorial. Possible mechanisms include weight-gain associated insulin resistance, $5\text{-}HT_{1A}$-antagonist-mediated hypoinsulinemia, and one or both of the aforementioned effects in those predisposed to the disease because of race or other genetic/environmental factors.

Dyslipidemia — Although the etiology of dyslipidemia is unknown, it is presumably related to weight gain and insulin resistance, factors also associated with the metabolic syndrome.

Hyperprolactinemia — The antidopaminergic activity of the atypical antipsychotics can remove the tonic dopamine-induced inhibition of prolactin secretion by the pituitary.

QTc prolongation — The QTc segment of the ECG reflects the repolarization phase of the cardiac cycle. Atypical antipsychotics and a number of other medications, as well as acquired and inherited disorders, can prolong repolarization; this effect is reflected in a prolonged QTc interval.[21] Prolongation of repolarization can be accompanied by spatial dispersion of repolarization. As a result, individual cardiac muscle fibers become responsive to electrical impulses at different times.

Neuroleptic malignant syndrome (NMS) — Manifestations of NMS are believed to be due to either blockade of dopaminergic receptors or withdrawal of exogenous dopaminergic agonists. Therefore, its probability is directly related to the antidopaminergic activity of the antipsychotic agent.

Figure 12.8 Management of AAP Side Effects

Clinical Considerations	Treatment Recommendations
Weight Gain	
Most AAPs are associated with significant weight gain. Clozapine and olanzapine appear to induce the most weight gain. Some evidence suggests that the weight plateau differs among agents and may stabilize within the first few months. There does not appear to be a clear correlation between weight gain and medication dose or severity of disease.	• Weigh patients at each visit and question about an increase in clothes or belt size. • Educate regarding dietary/physical activity. • Follow monitoring guidelines.
Dyslipidemia	
• Patients can develop hypertriglyceridemia.[21] • There are reported increases in serum triglycerides of $\geq$ 10–50%. • Most reports associate clozapine or olanzapine with dyslipidemia plus more significant weight gain/glucose intolerance.	• Since hypertriglyceridemia is an independent risk factor for coronary heart disease, lipid monitoring is important.
Hyperprolactinemia	
• Antidopaminergic activity can remove the tonic dopamine-induced inhibition of prolactin secretion by the pituitary; most common with risperidone and may or may not be symptomatic.[21] • Clinical manifestations include galactorrhea, gynecomastia, amenorrhea, anovulation, impaired spermatogenesis, decreased libido, anorgasmia, and impotence. • Routine screening is not indicated.	• Ask about symptoms during follow-up exams and assay prolactin levels if symptomatic; treat if elevated. • Treatment with dopaminergic agonists (e.g., bromocriptine) can worsen the psychiatric disorder; the best approach is usually to switch to another AAP.

(continued)

INTRODUCTION

PRESENTATION

CLINICAL PROCESS

PHARMACOTHERAPY

RESOURCES

Figure 12.8 (continued)

Clinical Considerations	Treatment Recommendations
QTc Prolongation	
• AAPs, other medications, and acquired/ inherited disorders can prolong repolarization, which is reflected in prolonged QTc interval.[21] • Consequences include arrhythmias (e.g., ventricular tachycardia, torsades de pointes). • The risk of torsades de pointes increases when the QTc interval > 500 ms. • The risk of arrhythmias increases with other metabolic abnormalities (e.g., hypokalemia or hypomagnesemia).	• Obtain baseline ECG, electrolytes, and renal/hepatic function tests when starting patients on ziprasidone, if patients are at risk. • Correct electrolyte abnormalities, discontinue non-essential medications that may also prolong interval; or use a substitute agent.
Neuroleptic Malignant Syndrome	
• An idiosyncratic reaction to antipsychotic agents. Risk factors may include agitation, dehydration, and IM administration (e.g., typical antipsychotics). • Manifested by hyperthermia, muscle rigidity, altered mental status, tremors, and manifestations of autonomic dysfunction (e.g., blood pressure lability, cardiac arrhythmias, and diaphoresis). • Usually occurs within several days of onset of therapy with drug levels within the therapeutic range. • Untreated, the course may be complicated by myocardial infarction, respiratory failure, mixed respiratory and metabolic acidosis, rhabdomyolysis, and acute renal failure.	• Treatment consists of rapid cooling with fluid and electrolyte support. • If the patient does not respond to cooling measures, bromocriptine (a dopamine antagonist) or dantrolene (a calcium-blocking skeletal muscle relaxant) may be required. • Antipyretics are not indicated.

Six atypical antipsychotics are now commercially available: clozapine, olanzapine, quetiapine, risperidone, ziprasidone, and aripiprazole. These atypical antipsychotics share many pharmacodynamic and pharmacokinetic properties.

Clozapine

Pharmacology — Clozapine has a complex receptor profile, including dopaminergic and serotonergic, as well as some muscarinic, histaminic, and adrenergic, activity. The dual action of activity at dopaminergic and serotonergic receptors is what led to the explosion of AAP development. Prior to clozapine, the older generation antipsychotic development activity focused on dopamine receptors only. Clozapine's serotonergic activity led to a major reconceptualization in the field.

Clozapine was the first atypical antipsychotic. Although a useful agent, the side effect and associated incidence of agranulocytosis make it impractical as a first-line agent for most patients. This medication, however, is an important second-line agent for patients who have failed other atypical antipsychotics or are treatment-resistant.

Clinical Trial Results — A randomized trial comparing clozapine with chlorpromazine in hospitalized patients with acute mania reported no significant differences in efficacy between the two drugs, although the trial was insufficiently powered to detect a difference at study endpoint.[22] However, results did suggest that clozapine may have a more rapid onset of action. In an uncontrolled trial for treatment-resistant mania, clozapine was efficacious.[23]

Administration — On the first day of treatment, one or two 25-mg tablets are usually administered with the initial oral dose not to exceed 75 mg. If well tolerated, the dosage may be increased daily in increments of 25–50 mg, so that a target dose of 300–450 mg/d is reached by the end of two weeks. In maintenance, long-term daily dosage ranges from 75–450 mg/d.[24]

Olanzapine

Pharmacology — Olanzapine has complex receptor activities with serotonergic and dopaminergic, as well as muscarinic, histaminic, and alpha adrenergic, activity.

Olanzapine is the most extensively studied of the atypical antipsychotics in patients with acute mania. It was the first atypical antipsychotic to receive FDA approval for this indication. When it was approved, it was redesignated as a psychotropic drug by the FDA as an attempt to describe its activity outside of psychotic disorders.

Clinical Trial Results — The efficacy of olanzapine for acute bipolar mania has been established in at least six randomized clinical trials.[25] Its efficacy has been established versus placebo, divalproex, and haloperidol. The drug was superior to placebo, at least as effective as divalproex, and comparable to haloperidol without associated worsening of depressive symptom scores during mania. The intramuscular preparation has been shown to be effective in the management of agitation in patients with acute bipolar mania.

Administration — When administered in combination with lithium or valproate, olanzapine therapy for acute bipolar mania should generally be started at 10 mg/d. In studies of short-term therapy, antimanic efficacy was present in a dose range of 5–20 mg/d.

Quetiapine

Pharmacology — Quetiapine has receptor activity at serotonergic, dopaminergic, and, to a lesser degree, at alpha-adrenergic and histaminic receptors.

Clinical Trial Results — Four randomized, controlled trials have demonstrated that quetiapine exerts antimanic activity.[25] As monotherapy, it is superior to placebo for acute mania symptom control. Similarly, quetiapine in combination with lithium or divalproex was superior to placebo in reducing manic symptoms. Additionally, patients enjoyed sustained antimanic effects at week 12 of therapy.[26]

Administration — In three of the four clinical trials referenced above, quetiapine was given in increasing doses of 100 mg/d for the first four days, followed by 600 mg/d on day five and 800 mg/d on day six. The average dose in responders was approximately 600 mg/d in divided doses in both the monotherapy and adjunct therapy trials.[26]

Risperidone

Pharmacology — Risperidone differs from the other atypical antipsychotics in that the drug has a relatively greater affinity for dopaminergic terminals than do the other agents. This effect is manifested in a dose-dependent manner in a tuberoinfundibular dopaminergic pathway by associated hyperprolactinemia.

Clinical Trial Results — Placebo-controlled trials of risperidone and haloperidol indicate that both medications, when combined with lithium, divalproex, or carbamazepine are superior to placebo and equally efficacious.[27–31] In addition, in studies using conventional doses, treatment with risperidone was accompanied by fewer extrapyramidal symptoms than was treatment with haloperidol.[25] Two of the placebo-controlled monotherapy trials cited also demonstrated the efficacy of risperidone in acute bipolar mania.

Administration — In patients with acute bipolar mania, risperidone can be administered once a day, starting with 2–3 mg/d. The dose can be then adjusted in increments of 1 mg/d. Antimanic activity is reported to be present in the 1–6 mg/d range, with usual antimanic dose of 4–6 mg/d.

Ziprasidone

Pharmacology — Ziprasidone has a mechanism similar to that of other atypical antipsychotics, but produces more extensive blockade of the serotonergic receptors. It also appears to block the serotonin and norepinephrine transporters to some degree. Because ziprasidone may produce QTc prolongation, there exists a risk of arrhythmia (including torsades de pointes) for patients taking this agent with other drugs that significantly prolong the QT interval, or

INTRODUCTION

PRESENTATION

CLINICAL PROCESS

PHARMACOTHERAPY

RESOURCES

in the presence of metabolic abnormalities that may cause QTc prolongation.

Clinical Trial Results — In one randomized, placebo-controlled study of ziprasidone monotherapy for patients with acute bipolar mania, the drug was significantly superior to placebo in symptom reduction, had a rapid onset of action, and had comparable tolerability to placebo.[32] A later study replicated these results and found that the drug also improved global illness severity in inpatients with acute bipolar mania (both manic and mixed episodes).[33]

Administration — Oral ziprasidone should be started at an initial, twice-daily dose of 40–60 mg taken with food. The daily dosage may subsequently be adjusted at intervals of at least one day, up to 80 mg twice a day, on the basis of the patient's individual clinical status.

Aripiprazole

Pharmacology — Aripiprazole is a newer atypical anti-psychotic. Its mechanism of action is as a partial dopamine D_2 agonist.

Clinical Trial Results — In studies of patients with acute mania, aripiprazole had superior efficacy compared with placebo and was at least as effective as haloperidol, without the latter's associated extrapyramidal adverse effects.[25]

Dosage Selection — Aripiprazole is administered at a starting dose of 15–30 mg/d for patients with acute mania. Maintenance and outpatient dosage may be lower.

Lamotrigine and Topiramate

Chapter 13 includes a detailed review of lamotrigine (pages 250 through 253) and topiramate (pages 253 through 254).

Antimanic Combination Therapy

To date, most of the accumulated data about antimanic combination therapy come from studies of lithium, valproate, and olanzapine. At present, lithium and/or valproate have been studied in combination with haloperidol, olanzapine, risperidone, quetiapine, or ziprasidone.[1] Although trials have not addressed dosing issues of monotherapy versus combination therapy, no data suggest that the standard doses should be adjusted when mood stabilizers of different classes are given in combination for acute episodes.

Recently, one small study examined long-term combination therapy using lithium and carbamazepine in 46 patients diagnosed with bipolar I disorder. That study found that, although adverse effects were marked, combining lithium with carbamazepine yielded substantial benefits over monotherapy.[34]

Treatment with two mood-stabilizing agents has been demonstrated to have a more rapid onset of action and greater efficacy than monotherapy in patients with acute bipolar mania.[1, 35, 36] Although there have been no randomized controlled trials, anecdotal reports suggest that the combination of lithium plus valproate is more efficacious than monotherapy with either agent.[37]

Studies have demonstrated that combination therapy is particularly valuable in patients with severe symptoms or psychotic features.[5]

> *Antipsychotics are an intuitive choice for psychotic mania, but divalproex and lithium are also effective.*

The efficacy of lithium appears to be less robust in patients with **mixed episodes** (mania with a minimum of depressive symptoms.)[7] In contrast, studies support valproate, risperidone, ziprasidone, aripiprazole, and olanzapine as agents with comparable efficacy in both manic and mixed episodes.[2, 38] Of the other antimanic drugs, only carbamazepine has been reported to produce responses in patients with mixed episodes.[39]

INTRODUCTION

PRESENTATION

CLINICAL PROCESS

PHARMACOTHERAPY

RESOURCES

References for Chapter 12

1. Keck PE Jr, McElroy SL. Treatment of bipolar disorder. In: Nemeroff CB, Schatzberg AF et al., eds *Textbook of Psychopharmacology*. 3rd Edition. Washington, DC: American Psychiatric Publishing; 2004.

2. Swann AC, Bowden CL, Morris D, et al. Depression during mania: treatment response to lithium or divalproex. *Arch Gen Psychiatry*. 1997;54(1):37–42.

3. Goodman LS, Hardman JG, Limbird LE, et al. *Goodman & Gilman's the Pharmacological Basis of Therapeutics*. New York: McGraw-Hill; 2001.

4. Keck PE Jr, Strakowski SM, Hawkins JM, et al. A pilot study of rapid lithium administration in the treatment of acute mania. *Bipolar Disord*. 2001;3(2):68–72.

5. American Psychiatric Association. Practice guideline for the treatment of patients with bipolar disorder (revision). *Am J Psychiatry*. 2002;159(Suppl 4):1–50.

6. (A.) Isojarvi JI: Reproductive dysfunction in women with epilepsy. *Neurology*. 2003; 61(6 Suppl 2):S27-34 (B.) Joffe H. Hall JE, Cohen LS, et al. A putative relationship between valproic acid and polycystic ovarian syndrome: implications for treatment of women with seizure and bipolar disorders. *Harv Rev Psychiatry*. 2003;11(2):99-108. (C.) Meo R, Bilo L. Polycystic ovary syndrome and epilepsy: a review of the evidence. *Drugs*. 2003;63(12):1185–227.

7. Keck PE Jr. The management of acute mania. *Br Med J*. 2003; 327(7422):1002–3.

8. Vasudev K, Goswami U, Kohli K. Carbamazepine and valproate monotherapy: feasibility, relative safety and efficacy, and therapeutic drug monitoring in manic disorder. *Psychopharmacology* (Berl). 2000; 150(1):15–23.

9. Joffe H, Cohen LS, Suppes T, et al. Valproate is associated with new-onset oligoamenorrhea with hyperandrogenism in women with bipolar disorder. *Biol Psychiatry*. 2006;59:1078–86.

10. Hartong EGTM, Moleman P, Hoogduin CAL, et al. Prophylactic efficacy of lithium versus carbamazepine in treatment-naive bipolar patients. *J Clin Psychiatry*. 2003;64:144–51.

11. Kleindienst N, Greil W. Differential efficacy of lithium and carbamazepine in the prophylaxis of bipolar disorder: results of the MAP Study. *Neuropsychobiology*. 2000;42(Suppl 1):2–10.

12. Moller HJ, Nasrallah HA. Treatment of bipolar disorder. *J Clin Psychiatry*. 2003;64 (Suppl 6):9–17; discussion 28.

13. Simpson GM, Glick ID, Weiden PJ, et al. Randomized, controlled, double-blind comparison of the efficacy and tolerability of ziprasidone and olanzapine in acutely ill patients with schizophrenia and schizoaffective disorder. *Am J Psychiatry*. 2004;161:1837–47.

14. Hirschfeld RMA, Keck PE Jr, Kramer M, et al. Rapid antimanic effect of risperidone monotherapy: a 3-week multicenter, double-blind, placebo-controlled trial. *Am J Psychiatry.* 2004;161:1057–65.

15. Keck PE, Marcus R, Tourkodimitris S, et al. A placebo-controlled, double-blind study of the efficacy and safety of aripiprazole in patients with acute bipolar mania. *Am J Psychiatry.* 2003;160:1651–8.

16. Turrone P, Kapur S, Seeman MV. Elevation of prolactin levels by atypical antipsychotics. *Am J Psychiatry.* 2002;159:133–5.

17. Gupta S, Masand P. Aripiprazole: review of its pharmacology and therapeutic use in psychiatric disorders. *Ann Clin Psychiatry.* 2004;16:155–66.

18. Daniel DG. Tolerability of ziprasidone: an expanding perspective. *J Clin Psychiatry.* 2003; 64,(Suppl 19):40–9.

19. Nasrallah HA, Tandon R. Efficacy, safety and tolerability of quetiapine in patients with schizophrenia. *J Clin Psychiatry.* 2002;63(Suppl 13):12–20.

20. Conley RR, Meltzer HY. Adverse events related to olanzapine. *J Clin Psychiatry.* 2000;61(Suppl 8):26–9.

21. Wirshing DA, Pierre JM, Erhart SM, et al. Understanding the new and evolving profile of adverse drug effects in schizophrenia. *Psychiatr Clin North Am.* 2003;26(1):165–90.

22. Barbini B, Scherillo P, Benedetti F, et al. Response to clozapine in acute mania is more rapid than that of chlorpromazine. *Int Clin Psychopharmacol.* 1997;12(2):109–12.

23. Calabrese JR, Kimmel SE, Woyshville MJ, et al. Clozapine for treatment-refractory mania. *Am J of Psychiatry.* 1996;153(6):759–64.

24. Fehr B, Ozcan M, Suppes T. Low doses of clozapine may stabilize treatment-resistant bipolar patients. *Archives of European Psychiatry.* 2005 Feb; 255(1):10–4. Epub 2004 Nov 12.

25. Keck PE Jr, McElroy SL. Second generation antipsychotics in the treatment of bipolar disorder; In press.

26. Sachs G, Chengappa KN, Suppes T, et al. Quetiapine with lithium or divalproex for the treatment of bipolar mania: a randomized, double-blind, placebo-controlled study. *Bipolar Disord.* 2004;6(3):213–24.

27. Khanna S, Victa E, Lyons B, et al. Risperidone in the treatment of acute mania: a double-blind, placebo-controlled study of 290 patients. *Br J Psychiatry*; 2005 Sep; 187:229–34.

28. Hirschfeld RM, Keck PE Jr, Kramer M, et al. Rapid antimanic effect of risperidone monotherapy: a 3-week multicenter, double-blind, placebo-controlled trial. *Am J Psychiatry.* 2004;161(6):1057–65.

29. Smulevich AB, Khanna S, Eerdekens M, et al. Acute and continuation risperidone monotherapy in bipolar mania: a 3-week placebo-controlled trial followed by a 9-week double-blind trial of risperidone and haloperidol. *Eur Neuropsychopharmacol.* 2005 Jan;15(1):75–84.

INTRODUCTION

PRESENTATION

CLINICAL PROCESS

PHARMACOTHERAPY

RESOURCES

30. Sachs GS, Grossman F, Ghaemi SN, et al. Combination of a mood stabilizer with risperidone or haloperidol for treatment of acute mania: a double-blind, placebo-controlled comparison of efficacy and safety. *Am J Psychiatry.* 2002;159:1146–54.

31. Yatham LN, Grossman F, Augustyns I, et al. Mood stabilisers plus risperidone or placebo in the treatment of acute mania. International, double-blind, randomised controlled trial. *Br J Psychiatry.* 2003;182:141–7.

32. Keck PE Jr, Versiani M, Potkin S, et al. Ziprasidone in the treatment of actue bipolar mania: a three-week, placebo-controlled, double-blind, randomized trial. *Am J Psychiatry.* 2003;160(4):741–8.

33. Potkin SG, Keck PE Jr, Segal S, et al. Ziprasidone in acute bipolar mania: a 21-day randomized, double-blind, placebo-controlled replication trial. *J Clin Psychopharmacol.* 2005;2(4):301–10.

34. Baethge C, Baldessarini RJ, Mathiske-Schmidt K, et al. Long-term combination therapy versus monotherapy with lithium and carbamazepine in 46 bipolar I patients. *J Clin Psychiatry.* 2005;66:174–82.

35. Müller-Oerlinghausen B, Retzow A, Henn FA, et al., for the European Valproate Mania Study Group. Valproate as an adjunct to neuroleptic medication for the treatment of acute episodes of mania: a prospective, randomized, double-blind, placebo-controlled, multicenter study. *J Clin Psychopharmacol.* 2000;20(2):195–203.

36. Tohen M, Chengappa KN, Suppes T, et al. Efficacy of olanzapine in combination with valproate or lithium in the treatment of mania in patients partially nonresponsive to valproate or lithium monotherapy. *Arch Gen Psychiatry.* 2002;59(1):62–9.

37. Freeman MP, Stoll AL. Mood stabilizer combinations: a review of safety and efficacy. *Am J Psychiatry.* 1998;155(1):12–21.

38. Tohen M, Jacobs TG, Grundy SL, et al., for the Olanzipine HGGW Study Group. Efficacy of olanzapine in acute bipolar mania: a double-blind, placebo-controlled study. *Arch Gen Psychiatry.* 2000;57(9):841–9.

39. Post RM, Uhde TW, Roy-Byrne PP, et al. Correlates of antimanic response to carbamazepine. *Psychiatry Res.* 1987;21(1):71–83.

Chapter 13: Antidepressants

Mood stabilizers, some anticonvulsants, atypical antipsychotics, and antidepressant agents are used in the treatment of patients with acute bipolar depression. This chapter discusses different classes of drugs related to the treatment of bipolar depression.

> *The primary goal of therapy with these agents is to ameliorate acute depressive symptoms without inducing manic, hypomanic, or mixed symptoms or episodes.*

Several different classes of medication have been used to treat symptoms of acute bipolar depression. These include lithium, anticonvulsants, atypical antipsychotics (newer generation psychotropics), selective serotonin reuptake inhibitors (SSRIs), bupropion, venlafaxine, duloxetine, tricyclic antidepressants (TCAs), and monoamine oxidase inhibitors (MAOIs). The mechanisms of action of these classes of agents differ considerably from each other, even within the same class. While various agents have similar efficacy, each agent with antidepressant action has its own advantages and disadvantages.

Based on clinical trial results, the American Psychiatric Association (APA) Guidelines recommend lithium and the anticonvulsant lamotrigine as first-line therapy for acute bipolar depression.[1] Valproate, carbamazepine, and topiramate are other anticonvulsants being studied for the treatment of patients with acute bipolar depression.[1-3] Since publication of the APA Guidelines, both a combination of olanzapine and fluoxetine (Symbyax®), as well as quetiapine (Seroquel®), have received FDA indication for the treatment of acute bipolar depression.

> *At the end of 2006, there are only two agents (one a combination) that are specifically approved to treat bipolar depression.*

INTRODUCTION

PRESENTATION

CLINICAL PROCESS

PHARMACOTHERAPY

RESOURCES

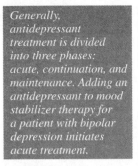

Generally, antidepressant treatment is divided into three phases: acute, continuation, and maintenance. Adding an antidepressant to mood stabilizer therapy for a patient with bipolar depression initiates acute treatment.

Selective serotonin reuptake inhibitors (SSRIs) are often prescribed for patients with both unipolar and bipolar depression. They are generally preferred to MAOIs and TCAs because of their tolerability and favorable side-effect profiles. Of the SSRIs, fluoxetine, paroxetine, and citalopram have been found to be effective for the treatment of acute bipolar depression **when combined with a mood stabilizer**.[4–6] These medications were considered first-line treatments (because of their favorable side-effect profile) until more recent information on other classes of agents became available.

Since the introduction of SSRIs, TCAs (e.g. imipramine and amitriptyline), and MAOIs (e.g., tranylcypromine), and other antidepressants like venlafaxine are considered second- or third-line agents, although they may be preferred in individual cases (see the latest TIMA guideline on page 157). Bupropion may be associated with less risk of manic/hypomanic switches.[7] Venlafaxine may pose greater risks of this type.[7]

Figure 13.1, on the next page, provides an overview of dose range and administration schedule for common antidepressant agents used to treat bipolar disorder. Material following this table covers clinical trial results, pharmacology, drug interactions, side effects, contraindications, and administration issues for these agents.

Figure 13.1 Antidepressant Agent Administration

Antidepressant Agent (class/medications)		Dose Range*	Admin. Schedule
	Lithium	0.6/1.0–1.2 mEq/L	BID or QHS
Anti-convulsants	Divalproex, valproate, valproic acid	80–125 µg/mL (acute) 50–125 µg/mL (overall)	BID or QHS
	Carbamazepine ER	400–1600 (4–12 µg/mL)	BID or QD
	Lamotrigine	50–200 mg/d**	QD
Atypical Anti-psychotics	Olanzapine***	10–20 mg/d	QHS
	Quetiapine	300–600 mg/d	QHS
SSRIs	Fluoxetine***	20–80 mg/d	QD
	Paroxetine	10–40 mg/d	QD
	Citalopram	10–40 mg/d	QD
	Fluvoxamine	100–400 mg/d	QD
Other Anti-depressants	Venlafaxine XR	75–350 mg/d	QD
	Bupropion	150–400 mg/d	QD
	Duloxetine	30–120 mg/d	QD
Tricyclic Anti-depressants	Amitriptyline	25–100 mg/d	QD
	Imipramine	100–300 mg/d	QD
MAOIs	Tranylcypromine	30–90 mg/d	BID

*Doses used for maintenance therapy may be lower.

**See product prescribing information.

***For the olanzapine-fluoxetine combination, see package insert/Physicians' Desk Reference.

Lithium

Because of clinical trial results over four decades, lithium is recommended as first-line therapy for the treatment of acute bipolar depression by the APA guidelines (by definition).[1]

Clinical Trial Results

Early trials in the 1960s of lithium in patients with acute bipolar depression reported that lithium was superior in efficacy to placebo: Thirty-six percent of patients had an unequivocal response and 79 percent had at least partial benefit.[8] In recent studies, patients with lithium levels below 0.8 mEq/L benefited from a combination of lithium and paroxetine. Above these lithium levels, however, there were no added antidepressant benefits from the addition of paroxetine or imipramine in this trial.[9] Thus, other antidepressants may not be required in patients with acute bipolar depression treated with lithium unless the patient cannot tolerate full lithium therapy. Young et al. compared combination therapy with lithium plus valproate to monotherapy with either drug plus paroxetine.[10] While the two regimens had equivalent efficacy, the combination mood-stabilizer regimen was not as well tolerated as monotherapy plus an antidepressant.

Anticonvulsants

Lamotrigine

Lamotrigine, along with lithium, is recommended by the APA guidelines as first-line therapy for acute bipolar depression. Lamotrigine is chemically unrelated to existing antiepileptic drugs.[11]

Clinical Trial Results

In a randomized, placebo-controlled, seven-week study of 195 patients with acute bipolar depression, treatment with lamotrigine at 50 mg/d and 200 mg/d was superior to placebo, and switch rates into hypomania or mania did not differ between groups.[11] Subsequently, the efficacy of lamotrigine in acute bipolar depression was confirmed in a parallel-group, flexible-dose study and in a double-blind crossover trial.[12, 13] Because lamotrigine appears to have no acute antimanic properties, many patients will also require a mood stabilizer, such as lithium.[14] A randomized, head-to-head comparison of lamotrigine with olanzapine-fluoxetine combination showed comparable efficacy for patients with bipolar I disorder experiencing depression.[15]

Pharmacology

Lamotrigine, in part, appears to exert its antiepileptic and antidepressant properties by modulating voltage-sensitive sodium channels and inhibiting the release of excitatory neurotransmitters.[16] After oral administration, the drug is rapidly absorbed and reaches peak plasma concentrations within 1.4–4.8 hours. When taken with meals, absorption is slightly delayed. Lamotrigine is approximately 55 percent bound to plasma proteins. Its volume of distribution is approximately one L/kg. With multiple doses, the medication's elimination half-life is approximately 26.4 hours.

Lamotrigine metabolism occurs predominantly by conjugation with glucuronic acid in the liver; approximately 70 percent is then excreted in the urine. Because metabolic and excretory pathways are hepatic and renal, lamotrigine should be administered cautiously in patients with liver and kidney disease. There are no significant age-related pharmacokinetic issues.

Drug Interactions

In patients also receiving valproate, the lamotrigine dose should be reduced by at least 50 percent to minimize potential toxicity and decrease the risk of a potentially serious rash. Valproic acid reduces the clearance of lamotrigine from the plasma and prolongs the drug's elimination half-life. As a result, lamotrigine levels are elevated approximately two-fold.[1]

Anticonvulsant drugs that upregulate hepatic drug-metabolizing activity, such as carbamazepine, increase plasma clearance and reduce lamotrigine's elimination half-life. With carbamazepine, the initial starting dose of lamotrigine is often doubled, and the target dose is higher. Oxcarbazepine does not affect the metabolism of lamotrigine to the same degree as carbamazepine. When combined with oxcarbazepine, the initial starting dose of lamotrigine should be the one used when no valproate or carbamazepine is used.

Side Effects

Common side effects associated with lamotrigine include:

- Neurologic changes: headache, dizziness, diplopia, ataxia
- Fatigue, asthenia, nausea, dry mouth
- Hypersensitivity reactions
- Cutaneous manifestations
- Rarely, Stevens-Johnson syndrome (toxic epidermal necrolysis), which is strongly associated with absolute starting dose and/or rate of initial titration.

Administration

> *If discontinuing lamotrigine for any reason for more than five days, it must be re-titrated from a starting dose amount.*

During the first two weeks, lamotrigine should usually be administered at a dose of 25 mg/d. The dose can then be doubled (50 mg/d) for weeks three and four. Thereafter, the dose can be increased in weekly increments of 50–100 mg/d to a maximum of 200–400 mg/d. To reduce the potential for a hypersensitivity reaction, lamotrigine should not be titrated

> *Following the recommended medication-dosing schedule is critical because of the rare risk of a medically serious rash (Stevens-Johnson syndrome, or toxic epidermal necrolysis).*

upward rapidly. In fact, slow titration appears to reduce the risk of serious rash in lamotrigine-treated patients to that observed with other antiepileptic drugs.[1] To decrease the likelihood of rash development, avoid initiating treatment immediately following a viral syndrome, or if the patient has recently come in contact with poison ivy/oak. Advise your patient not to use new chemicals (e.g., skin products or detergents) within eight weeks after lamotrigine treatment begins or after coming in contact with poison ivy/oak.

Divalproex/Valproate/Valproic Acid

There are no published, controlled trials of valproate or its various formulations in the treatment of acute bipolar depression. Thus, no recommendations can be made with regard to its use for this indication. Chapter 12 includes detailed information on valproate therapy on pages 226 through 229.

Carbamazepine

The principles behind carbamazepine therapy have been described in chapter 12. For dosage administration, side effects, and drug interactions, see pages 230 through 233 of that chapter.

Clinical Trial Results

In a small, double-blind, placebo-controlled crossover study, Ballenger et al. reported that 44 percent of patients with acute bipolar depression experienced a significant improvement from baseline with carbamazepine therapy.[17] In a more recent study, Dilsaver et al. demonstrated significant improvement in patients with acute bipolar depression treated with carbamazepine.[18] However, a subset of patients with mixed episodes has a poorer response to the medication.

Topiramate

Topiramate is a sulfamate-substituted monosaccharide. Although originally approved by the FDA for the treatment of partial seizures in adults, it has also been found to be useful in a number of non-seizure disorders. These include neuropathic pain, migraine, binge-eating, etc. There are no placebo-controlled trials of topiramate in the treatment of acute bipolar depression.[19] However, several trials suggest that it may be effective as an adjunctive measure.[20, 21]

Atypical Antipsychotics

Some atypical antipsychotics have been shown to have mood-stabilizing properties. Therefore, as a class, they might be anticipated to have efficacy in patients with acute bipolar depression. However, at present, only the olanzapine-fluoxetine combination and quetiapine are approved by the FDA for the treatment of bipolar depression.

> *Among atypical antipsychotics, randomized, controlled trials in acute bipolar depression have been completed only with olanzapine, quetiapine, and risperidone.*

Olanzapine

Tohen et al. conducted a double-blind, randomized, placebo-controlled, eight-week trial of olanzapine (5–20 mg/d) and olanzapine-fluoxetine combination (6 and 25 mg/d, 6 and 50 mg/d, and12 and 50 mg/d) versus placebo.[22] At eight weeks, the olanzapine, olanzapine-fluoxetine, and placebo groups demonstrated MADRS total scores lower than baseline by 15.0, 18.5, and 11.9, respectively.

Quetiapine

Recent research includes an eight-week, multicenter, double-blind, randomized, fixed-dose, placebo-controlled trial of quetiapine that focused on outpatients with bipolar I or II disorder (n = 511) experiencing a current episode of depression lasting at least four weeks. Those taking quetiapine (300 mg/d and 600 mg/d) monotherapy had lower-than-baseline MADRS total scores — 57 and 58 percent reductions (respectively) compared to the placebo group, which had a 36 percent reduction in scores.[23] A subsequent placebo-controlled acute depression study replicated the results in patients with bipolar I and II disorder.[24]

Risperidone

In a small, randomized, 12-week trial, Shelton et al. studied the effects of mood stabilizers in combination with adjunctive risperidone (1–6 mg/d) or paroxetine (20–40 mg/d), with similar doses of risperidone or paroxetine plus placebo, in patients with acute bipolar depression.[25] All three treatment groups showed similar reductions in MADRS scores.

Selective Serotonin Reuptake Inhibitors (SSRIs)

SSRIs are prescribed antidepressants that have efficacy in patients with both unipolar and bipolar depression. Their use along with a mood stabilizer is preferred to MAOIs and TCAs in many situations because of SSRIs tolerability and and favorable side-effect profile.

Clinical Trial Results

Of the SSRIs, fluoxetine, paroxetine, and citalopram have been studied and found to be effective as add-on therapy for the treatment of acute bipolar depression. The results suggest that patients with acute bipolar depression can be effectively treated with the combination of a mood stabilizer plus an SSRI. It is generally assumed that sertraline and fluvoxamine will show similar results; however, this has not been formally studied in bipolar depression.

In a study of 89 subjects with acute bipolar depression, treatment with fluoxetine produced improvement in 86 percent of patients.[5] This result was not only significantly better than placebo (p = 0.005) and the tricyclic antidepressant imipramine (p < 0.05), but significantly fewer fluoxetine-treated patients discontinued therapy because of adverse events. It should be noted that using the more modern analyses of intent-to-treat response rates with fluoxetine decreases the results to about 60 percent, and that some patients were also receiving lithium.

> *Like other antidepressants, SSRIs must be administered in conjunction with a mood stabilizer to prevent mood switches and cycle acceleration in patients with acute bipolar depression.*

INTRODUCTION

PRESENTATION

CLINICAL PROCESS

PHARMACOTHERAPY

RESOURCES

Paroxetine as an add-on therapy was compared with combination lithium and valproate in 27 patients randomized to paroxetine or a second mood stabilizer.[10] While improvements from baseline in Hamilton Depression Scale scores were significant and equivalent for both groups at week six ($p < 0.001$), more patients treated with lithium plus valproate dropped out of the trial. A second study confirmed the efficacy of paroxetine in lithium-treated patients, although efficacy over placebo was restricted to those with lithium levels less than 0.8 mEq/L.[4]

In an open, add-on treatment study of patients with bipolar I and II disorders, citalopram has also been reported to have efficacy in this indication.[6]

A recent search of *Medline* and related sources found no trials using sertraline or fluvoxamine. In clinical practice, sertraline is often one of the SSRIs of choice for bipolar depression treatment.[26] Leverich et al., however, looked at 159 patients with bipolar I and II disorders who received sertraline, venlafaxine, or bupropion as an add-on treatment in the acute and maintenance phases. They found a definite risk of mood switch when using these agents. The risk was highest when using venlafaxine and lowest in patients taking bupropion. Only 23 percent of patients who did not experience a threshold switch had a sustained antidepressant response in the maintenance phase.[7]

Pharmacology

Although the exact mechanism of action of SSRIs in depression is still somewhat unclear, three effects appear to contribute to the activity of the class:

1. Inhibition of neuronal reuptake of serotonin from the synaptic cleft
2. Desensitization of serotonergic feedback receptors
3. Downregulation of β-adrenergic receptors

Since clinical efficacy is often not seen for four to six weeks, the selective serotonin reuptake inhibition that occurs within hours is not solely responsible for the efficacy effect.

SSRIs are administered orally and are well absorbed from the gastrointestinal tract. Their half-life varies from 15 to 20 hours (fluvoxamine) up to 7 to 10 days (fluoxetine plus its active metabolites).[16] While the medication's elimination half-life does not affect efficacy or onset of action, it is an important consideration when the dose must be altered because of side effects or drug-to-drug interactions.

Side Effects

SSRI side effects relate to their effects on various neurotransmitters and receptors (see figure 13.2 on page 258).

Key considerations related to these side effects include:

- Adverse events in the GI tract are due to a combination of the medication's muscarinic and histaminergic blockade and activation of serotonergic receptors.
- Neurologic manifestations are secondary to blockade of the muscarinic and histaminergic receptors and to stimulation of the noradrenergic, serotonergic, and dopaminergic receptors.
- Cardiovascular side effects result from alpha-1-adrenergic blockade and activation of noradrenergic and dopaminergic receptors.

Drug Interactions

SSRIs are metabolized by hepatic cytochromes, principally CYP2D6 and CYP3A3/4. Consequently, there is the potential for drug interactions when they are co-administered with drugs that act as competitive inhibitors or inducers of various cytochromes. The prescribing information for each individual drug should be examined for potential side effects before an SSRI is prescribed.

Contraindications

Agents of this class should not be combined with MAOIs because of the risk of the serotonergic syndrome: confusion, tremor, myoclonus, hypertension, hyperthermia, and diarrhea. *Hypericum perforatum*, also known as St. John's Wort, is an herbal preparation with possible antidepressant

INTRODUCTION

PRESENTATION

CLINICAL PROCESS

PHARMACOTHERAPY

RESOURCES

properties and sold in extract form. Because of the herb's non-selective blockade of receptors, significant side effects, such as the serotonergic syndrome, can occur when patients are also receiving antidepressant therapy. In an attempt to manage symptoms, some patients may self-medicate with this herb, although its efficacy is not well demonstrated.

Figure 13.2 SSRI Side Effects in Relation to Their Effects on Neurotransmitter and Receptor Activity

Location of Side Effect	Symptoms	Receptor Activity
Gastro-intestinal	Dry mouth, constipation	Muscarinic blockade
	Weight gain	Histaminergic blockade
	Loss of appetite, nausea, vomiting, diarrhea	Serotonergic stimulation
Neurological	Blurred vision	Muscarinic blockade
	Sedation	Histaminergic blockade
	Anxiety, insomnia, tremor, diaphoresis	Noradrenegic stimulation
	Sexual dysfunction, akathisia, headache, insomnia	Serotonergic stimulation
	Agitation, psychosis	Dopaminergic stimulation
Cardio-vascular	Orthostatic hypotension	Alpha-1 adrenergic blockade
	Elevated blood pressure	Dopaminergic or noradrenergic stimulation
	Tachycardia	Noradrenegic stimulation

Other Antidepressants

Before the SSRIs and other alternative antidepressants were introduced, a tricyclic antidepressant (TCA) was the add-on drug of choice for the treatment of acute bipolar depression. However, TCAs are now generally considered second- or third-line agents for this indication.

Venlafaxine

Clinical Trial Results

In a study of venlafaxine and paroxetine in 60 women with acute bipolar depression treated with mood stabilizers, 48 percent of the patients treated with venlafaxine had a 50 percent or greater decrease in baseline Hamilton Depression Scale scores (p < 0.0001).[27] Although efficacy was equivalent to that produced by the SSRI, more patients treated with venlafaxine (13 vs. 3 percent) had a switch to hypomania or mania.

In the Leverich et al. study of those receiving either sertraline, venlafaxine, or bupropion as an add-on treatment in acute and maintenance phases, there was an increased risk of mood switch when using venlafaxine, where the ratio of threshold switches to subthreshold brief hypomanias was higher than with sertraline and bupropion in both the acute and continuation trials.[7]

Pharmacology

Venlafaxine is a phenethylamine bicyclic drug chemically unrelated to other antidepressants. It appears to potentiate CNS neurotransmitter activity through serotonin/norepinephrine reuptake inhibition. The drug is also a weak inhibitor of dopamine reuptake. Venlafaxine is rapidly absorbed after oral administration, metabolized in the liver by CYP2D6, and excreted in the urine. Consequently, its pharmacokinetic properties are extensively modified by the presence of hepatic and/or renal disease.

Side Effects

Side effects of venlafaxine include those typical of SSRIs and a risk of hypertension at higher doses.

INTRODUCTION

PRESENTATION

CLINICAL PROCESS

PHARMACOTHERAPY

RESOURCES

Bupropion

Clinical Trial Results

Results from the Leverich et al. research indicate a risk of mood switch when using bupropion and that, generally, only 23 percent of patients who did not experience a threshold switch had a sustained antidepressant response in the maintenance phase.[7]

Pharmacology

Bupropion is an aminoketone antidepressant chemically unrelated to other agents of this class. Although its exact mechanism of action is not precisely known, bupropion inhibits the neuronal uptake of both dopamine and norepinephrine. Experimentally, the medication acts as a stimulant and can cause seizures in large doses. The medication is rapidly absorbed after administration, metabolized and activated in the liver, and excreted in the urine.

Side Effects/Drug Interactions

Key considerations related to bupropion side effects include:

- Immediate-release bupropion in doses up to 450 mg/d induces seizures in approximately 0.4 percent (4 in 1000) of patients.

- The incidence of seizures in patients treated with extended-release bupropion is similar to that reported with SSRI treatment. The risk of seizures increases at doses over 450 mg/d in patients with epilepsy, bulimia nervosa, and head trauma. Bupropion levels can be elevated when co-administered with agents that interfere with its metabolism.

- Bupropion can produce agitation, insomnia, delusions, hallucinations, and weight loss.

- Bupropion induces hepatic cytochromes, and its metabolism can be affected by other drugs processed by the CYP450 system.

- Bupropion is generally safe for patients with cardiac disease.

- Bupropion is not significantly associated with the side effects of sexual dysfunction associated with SSRIs.

Bupropion induces hepatic cytochromes and can have its metabolism modified by other drugs processed by elements of the CYP450 system. The drug is generally safe in patients with cardiac disease and is not associated with the sexual dysfunction produced by the SSRIs. In patients with acute bipolar depression maintained on mood modifiers, treatment with bupropion was as effective as desipramine and less likely to precipitate a manic episode than was treatment with the TCA (11 vs. 30 percent).[28]

Duloxetine

Clinical Trial Results

There have been no published trials of duloxetine in bipolar depression. As with other antidepressants, treatment-emergent hypomania or mania must be considered a possibility with off-label use in bipolar patients.

Pharmacology

Duloxetine is a selective serotonin and norepinephrine reuptake inhibitor (SNRI) for oral administration. It is supplied in capsules containing enteric-coated pellets designed to prevent degradation of the drug in the acidic environment of the stomach; it is well absorbed after dosing. The elimination half-life is 12 hours (range 8 to 17 hours), and its pharmacokinetics are dose-proportional over the therapeutic range. Steady-state plasma concentrations are typically achieved after three days of dosing. Elimination of duloxetine is mainly through hepatic metabolism involving two P450 isoenzymes, CYP2D6 and CYP1A2. Duloxetine is a moderate inhibitor of CYP2D6 and does not induce CYP1A2 activity. Duloxetine metabolites are 70 percent and 30 percent excreted in the urine and feces, respectively.

Side Effects

Severe hepatic compromise is a contraindication for the use of duloxetine. The same is true in the case of severe renal compromise (creatinine clearance < 30 ml/min). Dose adjustment is not ordinarily required for patients with moderate renal compromise (creatinine clearance 30–80 ml/min). Transient 5 to 7 days, mild-to-moderate nausea in about one-third of patients is the most common adverse effect. Other adverse effects are similar to SSRIs, with the exception of sexual side effects in women, which were not different from placebo in registration trials. There are no dose-dependent effects on blood pressure.

Tricyclic Antidepressants (TCAs)

Clinical Trial Results

In general, treatment of acute bipolar depression with a TCA results in response rates that are superior to placebo and equivalent to or somewhat less effective than the comparators.[1] However, treatment with these drugs is accompanied by a higher rate of manic or hypomanic switch than treatment with other antidepressants. For example, in the study conducted by Nemeroff et al. of lithium plus paroxetine, six to 11 percent of patients treated with imipramine had a treatment-induced switch compared with only two and zero percent in the placebo and paroxetine-treated subjects, respectively.[4]

Pharmacology

Members of the TCA family share a chemical structure that contains at least two, joined benzene rings.[16]

Side Effects

Side effects result from the activity of the drugs as blockers of various receptors: muscarinic, histaminergic, and adrenergic. In general, TCAs that are secondary amines are less likely to produce anticholinergic and histaminergic adverse events.

Contraindications

The various TCAs are classified as class I antiarrhythmic medications. TCAs should often be avoided in patients with a history of heart disease and in individuals treated with other medications that can impair cardiac conduction (e.g., quinidine, procainamide), because TCA activity on cardiac sodium channels leads to a decrease in impulse propagation through the cardiac conduction system. Consequently, they can produce QTc prolongation, left bundle branch block, complete heart block, and/or sudden death.

Monoamine Oxidase Inhibitors (MAOIs)

Clinical Trial Results

MAOIs increase the concentration of monoamines at the synapse and appear to be superior to TCAs in their antidepressant activity in bipolar depression. Studies of the MAOI tranylcypromine demonstrated that it was more effective than imipramine. For example, compared with imipramine, patients with acute bipolar depression treated with tranylcypromine had significantly greater symptomatic improvement and global response rates, as well as lower attrition rates, than those who received the TCA.[29] The risk for developing mania is high when used without antimanic agents.[1, 8]

Pharmacology

Monoamine oxidase (MAO) catalyzes the oxidative degradation of monoamines, such as dopamine, serotonin, norepinephrine, and tyrosine. In the liver, MAO catabolizes monoamines from the gastrointestinal tract that are absorbed into the portal circulation.

> Because of safety issues, this group of medications is considered a second- or third-line choice for treatment of bipolar depression.

Side Effects

Side effects, which are due to inhibition of MAO activity, include postural hypotension, sexual dysfunction, insomnia, weight changes, and peripheral neuropathy; this last can often be prevented by the prophylactic administration of pyridoxine (vitamin B_6).

Toxicity

Inhibition of MAO in the liver is responsible for the systemic toxicity that can be observed with this class of drug. For example, patients treated with MAOIs who eat foods rich in monoamines can experience an adrenergic crisis that results in hypertension, tachycardia, arrhythmias, hyperpyrexia, and tremulousness. Hypertension in patients with severe adrenergic reactions can cause intracranial hemorrhage. The classic example of an adrenergic crisis occurs when a patient taking an MAOI attends a party and becomes severely symptomatic after ingesting red wine and strong or aged cheeses.

Treating Fatigue/Sedation Side Effects

Not only is fatigue a common symptom of depression, both unipolar and bipolar, but antidepressants typically cause some level of sedation that may be associated with adherence and overall quality of life issues. A number of studies have evaluated the efficacy of modafinil as augmentation treatment for these symptoms; these have found positive results.

Modafinil is FDA-approved for treating excessive sleepiness caused by narcolepsy or shift-work sleep disorder and for adjunctive use in treating obstructive sleep apnea/hypopnea syndrome. Modafinil is a "wake-promoting" central nervous system (CNS) stimulant that does not appear to affect the dopamine pathways associated with dependence and reward that are typical with other stimulants. Recent research indicates that modafinil significantly relieves symptoms of depression (especially fatigue and sleepiness) and the sedation effects of antidepressants.[30–33]

For patients with bipolar disorder, modafinil appears to be an effective medication for relieving symptoms of depression without the risk of mood switch. Nasr et al. recently completed a retrospective chart review of 191 patients and found no instance of medication-inducing manic/hypomanic switches. In addition, modafinil induced neither tolerance nor abuse among patients with or without a history of chemical abuse/dependence.[34] Additional research found that adjunctive modafinil given to patients with bipolar disorder in a dose of 100–200 mg daily improved residual depressive symptoms and fatigue without inducing manic destabilization.[35]

References for Chapter 13

1. American Psychiatric Association: Practice guideline for the treatment of patients with bipolar disorder (revision). *Am J Psychiatry.* 2002;159(Suppl 4):1–50.

2. Post RM, Uhde TW, Roy-Byrae PP, et al. Antidepressant effects of carbamazepine. *Am J Psychiatry.* 1986;43:29–34.

3. Small JG. Anticonvulsants in affective disorders. *Psychopharmacology Bulletin.* 1990;26:25–76.

4. Nemeroff CB, Evans DL, Gyulai L, et al. Double-blind, placebo-controlled comparison of imipramine and paroxetine in the treatment of bipolar depression. *Am J Psychiatry.* 2001;158(6):906–12.

5. Cohn JB, Collins G, Ashbrook E, et al. A comparison of fluoxetine imipramine and placebo in patients with bipolar depressive disorder. *Int Clin Psychopharmacol.* 1989;4(4):313–22.

6. Kupfer DJ, Chengappa KN, Gelenberg AJ, et al. Citalopram as adjunctive therapy in bipolar depression. *J Clin Psychiatry.* 2001;62(12):985–90.

7. Leverich GS, Altshuler LL, Frye MA, et al. Risk of switch in mood polarity to hypomania or mania in patients with bipolar depression during acute and continuation trials of venlafaxine, sertraline, and bupropion as adjuncts to mood stabilizers. *Am J Psychiatry.* 2006;163:232–9.

8. Zornberg GL, Pope HG, Jr. Treatment of depression in bipolar disorder: new directions for research. *J Clin Psychopharmacol.* 1993;13(6):397–408.

9. Nemeroff CB, Evans DL, Gyulai L, et al. Double-blind, placebo-controlled comparison of imipramine and paroxetine in the treatment of bipolar depression. *Am J Psychiatry.* 2001;158(6):906–12.

10. Young LT, Joffe RT, Robb JC, et al. Double-blind comparison of addition of a second mood stabilizer versus an antidepressant to an initial mood stabilizer for treatment of patients with bipolar depression. *Am J Psychiatry.* 2000;157(1):124–6.

11. Calabrese JR, Bowden CL, Sachs GS, et al. A double-blind placebo-controlled study of lamotrigine monotherapy in outpatients with bipolar I depression. Lamictal 602 Study Group. *J Clin Psychiatry.* 1999;60(2):79–88.

12. Bowden CL. Novel treatments for bipolar disorder. *Expert Opin Investig Drugs.* 2001;10(4):661–71.

13. Frye MA, Ketter TA, Kimbrell TA, et al. A placebo-controlled study of lamotrigine and gabapentin monotherapy in refractory mood disorders. *J Clin Psychopharmacol.* 2000;20(6):607–14.

14. Keck PE Jr, McElroy SL. Treatment of bipolar disorder. *Textbook of Psychopharmacology,* 3rd Edition. Nemeroff CB, Schatzberg AF, eds. American Psychiatric Publishing, Inc., Washington, DC, 2004.

15. Brown EB, McElroy SL, Keck PE Jr, et al. A 7-Week, Randomized double-blind trial of olanzapine/fluoxetine combination versus lamotrigine in the treatment of bipolar I depression. *J Clin Psychiatry.* 2006;67:1025–33.

16. Goodman LS, Hardman JG, Limbird LE, Gilman AG. *Goodman & Gilman's the pharmacological basis of therapeutics.* New York: McGraw-Hill; 2001.

17. Ballenger JC, Post RM. Carbamazepine in manic-depressive illness: a new treatment. *Am J Psychiatry.* 1980;137(7):782–90.

18. Dilsaver SC, Swann SC, Chen YW, et al. Treatment of bipolar depression with carbamazepine: results of an open study. *Biol Psychiatry.* 1996;40(9):935–7.

19. Suppes T. Review of the use of topiramate for treatment of bipolar disorders. *JClin Psychopharmacol.* 2002;22(6):599–609.

20. McIntyre RS, Mancini DA, McCann S, et al. Topiramate versus bupropion SR when added to mood stabilizer therapy for the depressive phase of bipolar disorder: a preliminary single-blind study. *Bipolar Disord.* 2002;4(3):207–13.

21. Hussein M. Treatment of bipolar depression with topiramate (abstract). *Eur Neuropsychopharmacol.* 1999;9(Suppl):S222.

22. Tohen M, Vieta E, Calabrese J, et al. Efficacy of olanzapine and olanzapine-fluoxetine combination int he treatment of bipolar I depression. *Archives of General Psychiatry.* 2003b:60:1079–88.

23. Calabrese JR, Keck PE Jr, Macfadden W, et al. A randomized, double-blind, placebo-controlled trial of quetiapine in the treatment of bipolar I or II depression. *Am J Psychiatry.* 2005;162:1351–1360.

24. Thase ME, Macfadden W, Weisler RH, et al. Efficacy of quetiapine monotherapy in bipolar I and II Depression: a confirmatory double-blind, placebo-controlled study (The BOLDER II Study). *J Clin Psychopharmacol.* 2006; in press.

25. Shelton RC, Addington S, Augenstein E, et al. Risperidone and paroxetine in bipolar disorder. In: *American Psychiatric Association Annual Meeting.* New Orleans, LA; 2001.

26. Gyulai I, Bowden CL, McElroy SL, et al. Maintenance efficacy of divalproex in the prevention of bipolar depression. *Neuropsychopharmacology.* 2003;28(7):1374–82.

27. Vieta E, Martinez-Aran A, Goikolea JM, et al. A randomized trial comparing paroxetine and venlafaxine in the treatment of bipolar depressed patients taking mood stabilizers. *J Clin Psychiatry.* 2002;63(6):508–12.

28. Sachs GS, Lafer B, Stoll AL, et al. A double-blind trial of bupropion versus desipramine for bipolar depression. *J Clin Psychiatry.* 1994;55(9):391–3.

29. Himmelhoch JM, Thase ME, Mallinger AG, et al. Tranylcypromine versus imipramine in anergic bipolar depression. *Am J Psychiatry.* 1991;148(7):910–6.

30. Price CS and Taylor FB. A retrospective chart review of the effects of modafinil on depression as monotherapy and as adjunctive therapy. *Depression and Anxiety.* 2005;21:149–53.

31. Schwartz TL, Azhar N, Cole K, et al. An open-label study of adjunctive modafinil in patients with sedation related to serotonergic antidepressant therapy. *J Clin Psychiatry* 2004;65:1223–27.

32. Fava M, Thase ME, DeBattista C. A multicenter, placebo-controlled study of modafinil augmentation in partial responders to selective serotonin reuptake inhibitors with persistent fatigue and sleepiness. *J Clin Psychiatry.* 2005;66:85–93.

33. Thase ME, Fava M, DeBattista C, et al. Modafinil augmentation of SSRI therapy in patients with major depressive dissorder and excessive sleepiness and fatigue: a 12-week, open-label, extension study. *CNS Spectr.* 2006 Feb;11(2):93–102.

34. Nasr S, Wendt B, Steiner K. Absence of mood switch with and tolerance to modafinil: a replication study from a large private practice. *J of Affective Disorders.* 2006 (in press).

35. Frye MA, Grunze H, Suppes T, et al. A Placebo-Controlled Evaluation of Adjunctive Modafinil in the Treatment of Bipolar Depression. Paper presented at the 44th Annual Meeting of the American College of Neuropsychopharmacology: Kona, Hawaii; December 16, 2005.

INTRODUCTION

PRESENTATION

CLINICAL PROCESS

PHARMACOTHERAPY

RESOURCES

Chapter 14:
Maintenance Medications

One of the most important long-term goals of therapy in patients with bipolar disorder is to prevent the recurrence, whether clinical or subclinical, of additional mood episodes. Approximately 90 percent of patients who experience a manic episode will have recurrent episodes, a fact that illustrates the need for adequate maintenance therapy. The other obvious long-term goal is to minimize ongoing symptoms.[1]

The efficacies of lithium, lamotrigine, and olanzapine in relapse prevention in bipolar I disorder have been demonstrated in placebo-controlled, long-term trials. Controlled trials of valproate, carbamazepine, clozapine, and aripiprazole also appear to show benefits for patients using these agents in the maintenance phase of bipolar disorder. Patients treated with a mood stabilizer plus an atypical antipsychotic also appear to have a lower risk of relapse if the combination is continued as maintenance treatment.

For general considerations in choosing the appropriate treatment for maintenance therapy, see page chapter 11.

Mood Stabilizers

This section reviews clinical trial results for medications used for maintenance treatment, including lithium, anti-convulsants, and atypical antipsychotics.

Lithium

Clinical Trial Results

Lithium is the best-studied and most-established agent for the maintenance therapy of patients with bipolar disorder. Placebo-controlled, randomized studies conducted in the 1960s and 1970s demonstrated that maintenance therapy with lithium provides a four-fold advantage compared with placeholder for preventing relapse at six- and 12-month intervals.[2] See page 271 for a description of recent 18-month, placebo-controlled lamotrigine trials.

For a full discussion of lithium, including side effects and dosing, refer to pages 221 through 226 in chapter 12.

Response Factors

When considering lithium maintenance therapy, it is important to consider factors that may reduce response to the drug (see figure 14.1, below).[3]

Figure 14.1   Factors that Impair Response to Lithium Maintenance Therapy[3]

- ◆ Rapid cycling
- ◆ Multiple prior mood episodes
- ◆ Absence of a family history of mood disorders
- ◆ Associated alcohol or substance use disorder
- ◆ Episode sequence of depression-mania-euthymia

From Bowden CL. Predictors of response to divalproex and lithium. *J Clin Psychiatr.* 1995;56(Suppl):25–30.

Maintaining Optimal Serum Lithium Levels

To maximize outcomes of lithium maintenance therapy, serum lithium levels usually need to be maintained at a level of 0.6–0.8 mEq/L or higher.[4] Several studies have demonstrated that lithium levels in the 0.4 mEq/L to 0.6 mEq/L range are associated with relapse rates and sub-syndromal manifestations that are 2.6-fold greater than those seen in patients with levels of 0.8 mEq/L or greater.[5, 6] Importantly, however, higher lithium levels are associated with greater toxicity and associated discontinuations. Therefore, the optimal serum lithium level in an individual patient is one that achieves the best efficacy-tolerability ratio.

Anticonvulsants — Clinical Trial Results

Valproate

Bowden et al. found that divalproex-treated patients (compared with patients in the placebo-controlled group), had lower rates of discontinuation for either a recurrent mood episode or depressive episode.[7]

Two open-label studies compared valproate with lithium as maintenance therapy in patients with bipolar disorder. In one study, both drugs had comparable efficacy, while in the other, the relapse rate of patients treated with the valpromide formulation of valproate was 20 percent lower than that of lithium after 18 months.[8, 9]

Lamotrigine

Two studies with similar designs evaluated the efficacy and tolerability of lamotrigine plus lithium for the prevention of mood episodes/relapses in outpatients with bipolar I disorder over a period of 18 months.[10, 11] Both lamotrigine and lithium were superior to placebo at prolonging the time to intervention for any mood episode. Lamotrigine was statistically superior to placebo at prolonging the time to intervention for a depressive episode, while lithium was statistically superior to placebo at prolonging the time to intervention for a manic or hypomanic episode.

For a full discussion of lamotrigine, including side effects and dosing, refer to pages 250 through 253 in chapter 13.

Carbamazepine

Because of methodological issues, the results of most studies of carbamazepine for the maintenance therapy of patients with bipolar disorder are often difficult to interpret. Two studies compared the drug with lithium. In the first study, relapse rates for carbamazepine and lithium did not significantly differ after one year (37 percent versus 31 percent, respectively).[12] However, results obtained in the

INTRODUCTION

PRESENTATION

CLINICAL PROCESS

PHARMACOTHERAPY

RESOURCES

trial's third year indicated that the combination of lithium and carbamazepine was superior to monotherapy with either drug.

In the second trial, however, carbamazepine was inferior to lithium at 2.5 years in a number of outcome measures; nevertheless, carbamazepine provided a superior benefit to patients with atypical symptoms.[13]

At this time, no study evidence exists on the relationship between serum carbamazepine levels and response rates.

Atypical Antipsychotics (Newer Generation Psychotropics) – Clinical Trial Results

Atypical antipsychotics provide a favorable risk-benefit profile in the treatment of acute bipolar disorder relative to the older typical antipsychotics. They are particularly useful when the episode is severe or when it is accompanied by psychotic manifestations. Evolving evidence suggests that these agents may have a role in long-term therapy of patients with bipolar disorder.

The clinical trial results described for the following medications represent completed controlled maintenance or prophylactic trials. We can anticipate an increase in information in this area, as a number of controlled trials are underway in evaluating medications in this class.

For a full discussion of atypical antipsychotics, including side effects and dosing, refer to pages 242 through 233 in chapter 12.

Clozapine

Suppes et al. studied the efficacy of long-term clozapine use in 38 patients with treatment-resistant schizoaffective or bipolar disorder. This was a randomized, open-label study.[14] Patients received either clozapine add-on or treatment as usual (no clozapine) and were followed for one year. There were significant between-group differences on all clinical symptom scales except depression. Patients with bipolar I disorder without psychotic symptoms showed improvement similar to that of the entire clozapine-treated group. Patients receiving clozapine required lower doses for stabilization than those with schizoaffective illness.

Olanzapine

Based on clinical trial evidence, olanzapine has been approved by the FDA for maintenance therapy of bipolar disorder. One trial found that olanzapine-treated patients had significantly lower rates of manic relapse compared with lithium-treated patients.[15] Other studies found patients on olanzapine had less manic and depressive recurrence than did patients in the placebo group, and that olanzapine performed as well as divalproex in terms of rates of mania remission.[16, 17]

Aripiprazole

Keck et al. studied the long-term efficacy of aripiprazole in 161 patients with bipolar I disorder and a recent manic or mixed episode.[18] Patients who had been stabilized on aripiprazole were randomized to placebo or aripiprazole treatment for a 26-week maintenance phase. Aripiprazole significantly prolonged time to relapse in bipolar I patients whose most recent episode was manic or mixed. The number of relapses to any type episode was also significantly lower in the aripiprazole group.

Other Biological Treatments

Minimal evidence points toward the efficacy of prefrontal transcranial magnetic stimulation (rTMS) in the treatment of bipolar depression. Its efficacy as a maintenance treatment is unproven as well. One small study looked at rTMS as adjunctive therapy in seven patients with bipolar depression.[19] Based on these results, the authors suggested that weekly rTMS treatments, in combination with medication, may be effective as maintenance therapy. More research is needed in this area.

References for Chapter 14

1. Hopkins HS, Gelenberg AJ. Treatment of bipolar disorder: how far have we come? *Psychopharmacol Bull.* 1994;30(1):27–38.

2. Keck PE Jr, Welge JA, Strakowski SM, et al. Placebo effect in randomized, controlled maintenance studies of patients with bipolar disorder. *Biol Psychiatry.* 2000;47(8):756–61.

3. Bowden CL. Predictors of response to divalproex and lithium. *J Clin Psychiatr.* 1995;56(Suppl):25–30.

4. Baldessarini RJ, Tondo L, Hennen J, et al. Is lithium still worth using? An update of selected recent research. *Harv Rev Psychiatry.* 2002;10(2):59–75.

5. Gelenberg AJ, Kane JM, Keller MB, Lavori P, Rosenbaum JF, Cole K, Lavelle J. Comparison of standard and low serum levels of lithium for maintenance treatment of bipolar disorder. *N Engl J Med.* 1989;321(22):1489–93.

6. Keller MB, Lavori PW, Kane JM, et al. Subsyndromal symptoms in bipolar disorder. A comparison of standard and low serum levels of lithium. *Arch Gen Psychiatry.* 1992;49(5):371–6.

7. Bowden CL, Calabrese JR, McElroy SL, et al. A randomized, placebo-controlled 12-month trial of divalproex and lithium in treatment of outpatients with bipolar I disorder. Divalproex Maintenance Study Group. *Arch Gen Psychiatry.* 2000;57(5):481–9.

8. Revicki D, Hirschfeld R, Keck PE Jr. Cost-effectiveness of divalproex sodium vs. lithium in long-term therapy for bipolar disorder. In: *American College of Neuropsychopharmacology Annual Meeting:* San Juan, PR; 1999.

9. Lambert P, Vernaud G. Comparative study of valpromide versus lithium as prophylactic treatment of affective disorders. *Nervure J Psychiatrie.* 1982;4:1–9.

10. Bowden CL, Calabrese JR, Sachs G, et al. A placebo-controlled 18-month trial of lamotrigine and lithium maintenance treatment in recently manic or hypomanic patients with bipolar I disorder. *Arch Gen Psychiatry.* 2003;60(4):392–400.

11. Calabrese JR, Bowden CL, Sachs G. A placebo-controlled 18-month trial of lamotrigine and lithium maintenance treatment in recently depressed patients with bipolar I disorder. *J Clin Psychiatry.* 2003;64(9):1013–24.

12. Denicoff KD, Smith-Jackson EE, Disney ER, et al. Comparative prophylactic efficacy of lithium, carbamazepine, and the combination in bipolar disorder. *J Clin Psychiatry.* 1997;58(11):470–8.

13. Greil W, Ludwig-Mayerhofer W, Erazo N, et al. Lithium versus carbamazepine in the maintenance treatment of bipolar disorders — a randomised study. *J Affect Disord.* 1997;43(2):151–61.

14. Suppes T, Webb A, Paul B, et al. Clinical outcome in a randomized 1-year trial of clozapine versus treatment as usual for patients with treatment-resistant illness and a history of mania. *Am J Psychiatry.* 1999;156(8):1164–9.

15. Tohen M, Marneros A, Bowden C, et al. Olanzapine versus lithium in relapese prevention in bipolar disorder: a randomized double-blind controlled 12-week trial. *Abstracts of the New Clinical Drug Evaluation Unit Annual Meeting*: Boca Raton, FL; May 26-28, 2003.

16. Tohen M, Ketter TA, Zarate CA, et al. Olanzapine versus divalproex sodium for the treatment of acute mania and maintenance of remission: a 47-week study. *Am J Psychiatry.* 2003;160(7):1263–71.

17. Tohen B, Bowden C, Calabrese J, et al. Olanzapine's efficacy for relapse prevention in bipolar disorder: a placebo-controlled, randomized, double-blind controlled 12-month trial. In: *Abstracts of the Fifth International Conference on Bipolar Disorder*. Pittsburgh, PA; June 16, 2003.

18. Keck PE Jr, Sanchez R, Marcus RN, et al. Aripiprazole for relapse prevention in bipolar disorder in a 26-week trial. Presented at *The 157th Meeting of the American Psychiatric Association.* New York, NY; May 1-6, 2004a.

19. Li X, Nahas Z, Anderson B, et al. Can left prefrontal rTMS be used as a maintenance treatment for bipolar depression? *Depression and Anxiety.* 2004;20:98–100.

INTRODUCTION

PRESENTATION

CLINICAL PROCESS

PHARMACOTHERAPY

RESOURCES

Chapter 15: Assessment Tools

Using Structured Clinical Interviews

Highly structured diagnostic interviews typically reduce the emphasis on clinician judgment present in open-ended interviews. These tools may require specialized training to administer correctly and can be time-consuming. Clinical interviewing tools for diagnosing bipolar disorder include:

> *The benefit of structured clinical interviews is their ability to provide objective criteria for diagnostic decision making.*

- **The Schedule for Affective Disorders and Schizophrenia (SADS)** — Developed to differentiate between affective disorders and schizophrenia, the SADS must be administered by trained professionals. The instrument is a two-part, semi-structured interview that takes approximately 1.5 to 2 hours to administer. Questions are progressive and have built-in criteria for whether or not to rule out the symptoms for current diagnostic purposes.

- **Diagnostic Interview Schedule (DIS)** — The DIS is a highly structured, diagnostic interview designed to be administered by experienced lay interviewers without clinical training. It is designed to assess the prevalence of psychiatric disorders in the general population.[1] Other research supports interrater reliability when conducted by professionals and paraprofessionals.[2] The computerized version can be self administered with availability of an assistant to answer questions if needed.

- **The Structured Clinical Interview for the DSM-IV (SCID)** — The SCID is a structured, broad-spectrum instrument that adheres closely to the DSM-IV decision trees for psychiatric diagnosis.[3] There are multiple versions, including a briefer clinical version, research version, and a module to assess for the presence of personality disorders. The SCID is

SECTION E: RESOURCES FOR ASSESSMENT AND TREATMENT

designed for use by trained interviewers to ensure a structured and consistent format for investigating psychiatric symptoms.

Using Clinician–Administered Observational Rating Scales

A number of assessment tools exist that involve a combination of structured to semi-structured interview and behavioral observations. These tools were specifically designed for administration by an interviewer trained to mitigate interviewer bias and variations in the interview environment.

Those clinician-administered instruments commonly used with **manic symptoms** include the:

- **Young Mania Rating Scale (YMRS)** — This 11-item measure was designed to assess the severity of manic symptoms and to detect the effects of treatment on mania.[3] It includes both mild and severe versions of manic symptoms. Items are ranked on a scale of $0-4$ or $0-8$. Professionals can administer the YMRS after minimal training.

  The YMRS (typically utilized as the "gold standard" measurement of manic symptoms in research settings) and other observational rating scales serve an important educational role, helping primary care clinicians better understand and recognize mania.

  The YMRS has demonstrated good interrater and inter-item reliability and has a strong association to other measures of manic symptoms.[4]

- **The Bech–Rafaelsen Mania Scale (MAS)** — The MAS is a clinician-rated assessment tool for measuring mania symptoms in patients with bipolar disorder.[5] The 11-item scale assesses mania over a minimum of the three previous days, and covers major symptom domains, such as mood, speech patterns, sleep disturbance, increased activity, irritability, and grandiose delusions. Ratings are made on a four-point scale for each question, and scores are standardized such that scores less than 15 indicate hypomania, scores around 20 indicate moderate mania, and scores around 28 indicate severe mania. The MAS has been validated in adults and has been shown to have good responsiveness, detecting changes in mania symptoms in trials as short as one week.[6]

- **Clinician-Administered Rating Scale for Mania (CARS-M)** — The CARS-M was designed to evaluate the severity of manic and psychotic symptoms, and to detect changes in such symptoms over the course of treatment.[7] It includes two subscales that are individually scored, measuring mania and psychosis respectively. Items assessing mania were derived from the SADS, described previously. The scale includes 15 items that are rated from 0–6 on a Likert scale, except for one item, insight, which is rated 0–4. Each item has anchors, and the scale also includes prompts to aid clinicians in probing certain symptom domains. Clinicians are also permitted to use collateral information, such as family and medical histories, when making ratings.

Reliability for the CARS-M is substantial.[7] Additionally, the CARS-M correlates strongly (0.94) with the YMRS. Research evidence exists that the manic subscale can differentiate patients suffering from mania from those with other severe psychiatric disturbance.[6]

Those clinician-rated scales commonly used to assess **depressive symptoms** include the:

- **Hamilton Rating Scale for Depression (HAM-D)** — Historically, the HAM-D has been the most common interview method for assessing depression, initially created to assess depression severity in those already diagnosed.[8–10] The HAM-D is a 21-item scale completed during a 30-minute interview (only the first 17 items are scored, thus the scale is often referred to as the "HAM-17"). It includes a checklist of ranked items on a scale of 0–4 or 0–2. The HAM-D

INTRODUCTION

PRESENTATION

CLINICAL PROCESS

PHARMACOTHERAPY

RESOURCES

was designed to be administered by physicians, psychologists, and social workers experienced with psychiatric populations; however, it can be administered by non-clinicians after some training.

- **Montgomery-Äsberg Depression Rating Scale (MADRS)** — The MADRS is a clinician-rated measure, which provides data on overall depression severity and specific depressive symptoms.[11-13] It has been demonstrated to be sensitive to change in depression symptoms over time. The MADRS includes 10 items, which are rated on a scale of 0–6. Observations as well as verbal information are used in the ratings.

  The reliability of the MADRS is acceptable and comparable to other observer-rated depression scales, with joint reliability for the total scale ranging from 0.76–0.95. The following mean scores from the MADRS correlate with global severity measures from the DSM: very severe, 44; severe, 31; moderate, 25; mild, 15; and recovered, 7.[12]

- **Inventory of Depressive Symptomatology-Clinician Rated (IDS-C)** — This measure was designed to capture symptoms of depression in both inpatients and outpatients, and is derived from diagnostic criteria for major depressive disorder found in the DSM-IV.[14] It includes both a self-report (the IDS-SR described on page 285) and a clinician-rated form. The latter includes 30 items, which are scored on a four-point anchored scale. It includes a semi-structured interview to assist a trained clinician interviewer.

The IDS-C is unique in its efforts to be more comprehensive, including coverage of atypical and melancholic features as well as somatic and cognitive features of depression.

The IDS-C possesses excellent reliability, achieving an internal consistency of 0.94 in a large sample.[14] It is highly correlated with other depression rating scales. Recently, the Quick

Inventory of Depressive Symptomotology (QIDS), which consists of 16 questions from the IDS, has demonstrated reliability as well.[15] The QIDS is also available in clinician- and self-rated forms.

Using Self-Ratings

Self-ratings are completed independently by the patient and help detect the presence or absence of symptoms. Several self-report instruments serve as effective screening tools for determining patients who may be suffering from bipolar illness.

> At best, "red flag" scores on self-report instruments signal the need for more thorough clinical interviewing with patients as well as significant others in their lives.

It is important to keep in mind that a patient's level of insight into their symptoms can impact reliability. Thus, these measures serve best as educational tools for the physician to help make a diagnosis of major depressive disorder one in which the prospect of bipolar illness has been excluded. One tool useful for differential diagnosis is the Patient Health Questionnaire (PHQ-9), which was developed for assessing depression in the primary care setting. This tool, used along with other measures (e.g., the MDQ) and careful clinical interviewing, can help guide the clinician to differentiate major depression from depressive symptoms that are part of the bipolar spectrum.

Self-ratings used in **assessing possible bipolar illness** include the:

- **Patient Health Questionnaire (PHQ-9)**[16–18] — The PHQ-9 is a nine-question depression scale originally developed as part of Pfizer's PRIME-MD project. It is the instrument recommended by the MacArthur Initiative on Depression and Primary Care because of the strength of multiple validation studies in the primary care setting.

  The PHQ-9 is based directly on the diagnostic criteria for major depressive disorder in the DSM-IV. It has been shown to be useful in screening, diagnosis, and longitudinal follow-up. The MacArthur Initiative also recommends questioning chronicity to assist in treatment planning for those with mild but chronic impairment (e.g., "In the past two years, have you felt depressed or sad most days, even if you felt okay sometimes?").

A PHQ-9 score > 10 had a sensitivity of 88 percent and a specificity of 88 percent for major depression in validation studies. PHQ-9 scores of 5, 10, 15, and 20 represented mild, moderate, moderately severe, and severe depression, respectively. Patients in both traditional primary care and women in obstetrics-gynecology treatment settings had similar results. As in other self-report instruments, clinical judgment must be used in the interpretation of the results.

- **Beck Depression Inventory (BDI-2)**[19, 20] — The BDI-2 assesses depressive symptoms based on DSM-IV criteria. The patient is asked to respond to 21 items covering specific thoughts and feelings in the areas of cognitive, affective, somatic, and vegetative symptoms of depression experienced within the past week. It is useful for those 13 years and older and can be administered individually or in groups in a written or oral format. It takes approximately five to 10 minutes to complete and can be scored manually or by computer, with a computer-based interpretation of the scores available. The BDI-2 is intended to be a screening tool for depression, with particular attention to items on hopelessness and suicidal ideation as the best indicators of potential suicidality.[21, 22]

Self-ratings that **specifically screen for bipolar illness** include the:

- **Temperament Evaluation of Memphis, Pisa, Paris and San Diego Autoquestionnaire version (TEMPS-A)** — The TEMPS-A is a self-report questionnaire measuring different temperaments in both psychiatric and healthy populations. The clinical version consists of 50 self-report items, loading on four temperament factors (dysthymic, hyperthymic, cyclothymic, and irritable).[23] The short version consists of 39 self-report items, loading on five factors (dysthymic, hyperthymic, cyclothymic, irritable, and anxious).[24] Items are designed to measure stable traits, attitudes, and outlook of the patient, including energy level, emotional outlook, and mood reactivity. Both versions have been validated in adults and are scored manually.

> *The TEMPS-A is particularly useful in distinguishing bipolar I and II subtypes, with particular emphasis on the cyclothymia subscale of the questionnaire.[22]*

- **Bipolar Spectrum Diagnostic Scale (BSDS)** — Initially developed for clinician use, this tool is frequently used as a self-report tool to initiate conversations about bipolar spectrum symptoms between patients and their health care providers. The scale applies to the entire spectrum of bipolar disorders and presents a descriptive story that patients can respond to on a line-by-line basis if they identify with some element. The BSDS has been found to be highly sensitive and specific for bipolar spectrum illness.[25]

- **Internal State Scale (ISS)** — This 17-item, self-report scale assesses both manic and depressive symptoms and can be useful for identifying mixed states as well as classic mania and depression. Items are presented as a visual analog scale; respondents mark their response along the scale from 0 to 100. Factor analysis of the ISS reveals four subscales, called "Activation," "Perceived Conflict," "Well-Being," and "Depression." The ISS can be completed in approximately 15 to 20 minutes.

A multi-site, public sector sample validated the ISS' initial research clinic sample, confirming the ISS to be an effective discriminator of mood states in bipolar disorder. That study also validated that a revised scoring algorithm had made the ISS a feasible tool for formal identification of mixed episodes.[26]

• **Mood Disorder Questionnaire (MDQ)**[27] — This self-report diagnostic instrument is a brief, self-administered screening tool for bipolar disorder.[27] However, the MDQ provides little information about the severity and duration of symptoms.[27] It includes 13 "yes/no" items derived from both DSM-IV criteria and clinical experience. A positive screen requires that seven or more items must be endorsed, several of the items must co-occur, and the symptoms cause at least moderate psychosocial impairment.

The sensitivity and specificity of the MDQ have been debated and evaluated in recent years. Hirschfeld et al. found the MDQ's specificity to be 0.972, and its sensitivity to be 0.281 in the general population.[28] In 2004, Miller et al. found that, in general, the MDQ is of greater use with insightful patients, and those who have BD I, compared with BD II/NOS.[29] The difference in sensitivity between BD I and II was statistically significant. Overall, Miller's study found the MDQ had a sensitivity of 0.58, and a specificity of 0.67. In a family practice study of 649 patients treated for major depression, when the results were compared with the Structured Clinical Interview for the DSM-IV(TR), the sensitivity and specificity of the MDQ were 58 percent and 93 percent, respectively.[30]

Phelps and Ghaemi reviewed data from four studies (including the Hirschfeld and Miller studies), three of which evaluated the MDQ and one that evaluated the Bipolar Spectrum Diagnostic Scale (BSDS).[31] In addition to sensitivity and specificity, Phelps and Ghaemi also looked

This scale may be a useful adjunct to other assessments because it is brief and because patients can complete it independently in the waiting room. However, diagnostic decisions cannot be made based on the MDQ alone.

at the positive and negative predictive values (PPV and NPV) of the instruments, and factored in prior probabilities and the likely prevalence of bipolar disorder. They found that in the community setting (a typical primary care practice area), "clinicians' estimates of prior probability have as much, or in many cases more, impact on the clinical performance of the bipolar screening tools than the tests' sensitivity and specificity."

- **The Altman Mania Rating Scale (AMRS)**[32] — The AMRS is a five-item, patient self-rating mania scale, designed to assess the presence and/or severity of manic symptoms. The AMRS is designed to be a screening instrument, and a diagnosis cannot be reliably made based upon results from this tool. All items are scored from 0 (absent) to 4 (present to a severe degree), based on increasing severity. A cutoff score of 6 or higher on the AMRS indicates a high probability of a manic or hypomanic condition (based on a sensitivity rating of 85.5 percent and a specificity rating of 87.3 percent). A score of 5 or lower is less likely to be associated with significant symptoms of mania. A score of 6 or higher may indicate a need for treatment and/or further diagnostic workup (to confirm a diagnosis of mania or hypomania).

- **The IDS-SR**[14, 33] — This is a self-report companion scale to the IDS-C described on pages 280–281. It includes 30 multiple-choice items, with most scored from 0 (least severe) to 3 (most severe). Completion of the IDS-SR requires approximately 15–20 minutes, and adequate reading ability. The IDS-SR is highly correlated with other self-report measures of depression (0.93 with the BDI) and with its companion, clinician-rated version (0.91 with the IDS-C). The QIDS-SR (16 questions taken from the IDS) is also now validated and available.[15]

References for Chapter 15

1. Robins LN, Marcus L, Reich W, et al. *Diagnostic Interview Schedule, Version IV.* St. Louis, MO, Department of Psychiatry: Washington School of Medicine; 1996.

2. Helzer JE, Spitznagel EL, McEvoy L. The predictive validity of lay Diagnostic Interview schedule diagnosis in the general population. A comparison with physician examiners. *Arch Gen Psychiatry.* 1987;44(12):1069–77.

3. First MB, Spitzer RL, Gibbon M, et al. *Structured Clinical Interview for DSM-IV – Clinician Version (SCID-CV) (User's Guide and Interview).* Washington DC: American Psychiatric Press; 1997.

4. Young RC, Biggs JT, Ziegler BE, et al. A rating scale for mania: reliability, validity and sensitivity. *Br J Psychiatry.* 1978;133:429–35.

5. Bech P, Bolwig TG, Kramp P, et al. The Bech–Rafaelsen Mania Scale and the Hamilton Depression Scale. *Acta Psychiatrica Scandinavica.* 1979; 59:420–30.

6. Bech P. The Bech-Rafaelsen Mania Scale in clinical trials of therapies for bipolar disorder: a 20-year review of its use as an outcome measure. *CNS Drugs.* 2002;16(1):47–63.

7. Altman EG, Hedeker DR, Janicak PG, et al. The Clinician-Administered Rating Scale for Mania (CARS-M): development, reliability, and validity. *Biol Psychiatry.* 1994;36(2):124–34.

8. Hamilton M. A rating scale for depression. *J Neurol Neurosurg Psychiatry.* 1960;23:56–62.

9. Hamilton M. Development of a rating scale for primary depressive illness. *Br J Soc Clin Psychol.* 1967;6:278–96.

10. Williams JB. A structured interview guide for the Hamilton Depression Rating Scale. *Arch Gen Psychiatry.* 1988;45:742–47.

11. Montgomery SA, Äsberg M. A new depression scale designed to be sensitive to change. *Br J Psychiatry.* 1979;134:382–9.

12. Kearns NP, Cruickshank CA, McGuigan KJ, et al. A comparison of depression rating scales. *Br J Psychiatry.* 1982;141:45–9.

13. Davidson J, Turnbull CD, Strickland R, et al. The Montgomery-Äsberg Depression Scale: reliability and validity. *Acta Psychiatr Scand.* 1986; 73:544–8.

14. Rush AJ, Giles DE, Schlesser MA, et al. The Inventory for Depressive Symptomatology (IDS): preliminary findings. *Psychiatry Res.* 1986;18(1):65–87.

15. Rush AJ, Bernstein IH, Trivedi MH, et al. An evaluation of the Quick Inventory of Depressive Symptomatology and the Hamilton Rating Scale for depression: a sequenced treatment alternatives to relieve depression trial report. *Biolo Psychiatry.* 2006 Mar;59(6):493–501.

16. Spitzer R, Kroenke K, Williams J. Validation and utility of a self-report version of PRIME-MD: the PHQ Primary Care Study. *JAMA*. 1999;282:1737–44.

17. Kroenke K, Spitzer RL. The PHQ-9: A new depression and diagnostic severity measure. *Psychiatric Annals*. 2002;32:509–21.

18. Lowe B, Unutzer J, Callahan CM, et al. Monitoring depression treatment outcomes with the Patient Health Questionnaire-9. *Medical Care*. 2004;42(12): 1194–201.

19. Beck AT, Steer RA, Brown GK. *Beck Depression Inventory – Second Edition Manual*. San Antonio, TX: Psychological Corporation, Harcourt Brace; 1986.

20. Beck AT, Steer RA, Garbin MG. Psychometric properties of the Beck Depression Inventory: twenty-five years of evaluation. *Clin Psychol Rev*. 1988;8:77–100.

21. Carlson GA. Mania and ADHD: comorbidity or confusion. *J Affect Disord*. 1998 Nov;51(2):177–87.

22. Murphy LL, Impara JC, Plake, BS (eds). *Tests in print V*. Lincoln, NE: University of Nebraska Press; (1999).

23. Akiskal HS, Akiskal KK, Haykal RF, et al. TEMPS-A progress towards validation of a self-rated clinical version of the Temperament Evaluation of the Memphis, Pisa, Paris, and San Diego Autoquestionnaire. *J Affect Disord*. 2005a;85:3–16.

24. Akiskal HS, Mendlowicz MV, Jean-Louis G, et al. TEMPS-A validation of a short version of a self-rated instrument designed to measure variations in temperament. *J Affect Disord*. 2005b;85:45–52.

25. Nassir Ghaemi S, Miller CJ, Berv DA, et al. Sensitivity and specificity of a new bipolar spectrum diagnostic scale. *J Affect Disord*. 2005 Feb;84(2–3):273–7.

26. Bauer MS, Vojta C, Kinosian B, et al. The Internal State Scale: replication of its discriminating abilities in a multisite, public sector sample. *Bipolar Disord*. 2000 Dec;2(4):340–6.

27. Hirschfeld RM, Williams JB, Spitzer RL, et al: Development and validation of a screening instrument for bipolar spectrum disorder: the Mood Disorder Questionnaire. *Am J Psychiatry*. 2000;157:1873–5.

28. Hirschfeld RM, Holzer C, Calabrese JR, et al. Validity of the mood disorder questionnaire: a general population study. *Am J Psychiatry*. 2003;160:178–80.

29. Miller CJ, Klugmanc J, Bervc DA, et al. Sensitivity and specificity of the Mood Disorder Questionnaire for detecting bipolar disorder. *J Affect Disord*. 2004;81:167–71.

30. Hirschfeld RM, Cass AR, Holt DC, et al. Screening for bipolar disorder in patients treated for depression in a family medicine clinic. *J Am Board Fam Pract*. 2005 Jul-Aug;18(4):233–9.

INTRODUCTION

PRESENTATION

CLINICAL PROCESS

PHARMACOTHERAPY

RESOURCES

31. Phelps JR, Ghaemi SN. Improving the diagnosis of bipolar disorder: predictive value of screening tests. *J Affect Disord.* 2006;92:141–48.

32. Altman EG, Hedeker D, Peterson JL, et al. The Altman Self-Rating Mania Scale. *Biol Psychiatry.* 1997;42:948–55.

33. Rush AJ, Gullion CM, Basco MR, et al. The inventory of depressive symptomatology (IDS): psychometric properties. *Psychol Med.* 1996;26:477–86.

Chapter 16: Internet Resources

For Patients:

Child & Adolescent Bipolar Foundation
www.bpkids.org

This parent-led, Web-based support and advocacy organization helps families raising children and adolescents diagnosed with, or at risk for, early-onset bipolar disorder. Features include access to relevant research articles, instructional materials for parents and educators, on-line support groups and message boards, and directories of local support groups and trained treatment professionals.

Depression and Bipolar Support Alliance
www.dbsalliance.org

This non-profit support organization educates the public, healthcare professionals, and legislators about the diagnosis and treatment of bipolar disorder and depression. Web site features include information on support groups, programs and publications, resources, and state chapters.

National Alliance for the Mentally Ill (NAMI)
www.nami.org

NAMI is the nation's largest grassroots mental health organization serving people living with serious mental illness and their families. The NAMI Web site offers information about mental disorders as well as resources for education and advocacy.

schoolpsychiatry.org
www.schoolpsychiatry.org

This site provides information and resources for parents, educators, and clinicians regarding a wide range of mental health conditions in children and adolescents, with a focus on the school setting. The site is a joint project of the School

INTRODUCTION

PRESENTATION

CLINICAL PROCESS

PHARMACOTHERAPY

RESOURCES

Psychiatry Program and the Mood & Anxiety Disorders Institute Resource Center in the Massachusetts General Hospital Department of Psychiatry. In addition to offering information on child and adolescent bipolar disorder, the site provides diagnostic screening tools, describes commonly used psychological interventions (counseling) and medications, suggests accommodations for home and school, and includes an annotated listing of recommended Web sites for further reading.

For Healthcare Practitioners

The Mood and Anxiety Disorders Program (MAP)
http://intramural.nimh.nih.gov/mood/

This site, sponsored by the world's largest research program focused on mood and anxiety disorders presents information on research currently underway for bipolar disorder as well as depression and anxiety disorders.

Facts for Health
www.factsforhealth.org

Facts for Health was developed by the Madison (WI) Institute of Medicine to provide medical professionals and the general public with information about a variety of medical conditions, including premenstrual dysphoric disorder.

National Institute of Mental Health,
Health Information on Bipolar Disorder
www.nimh.nih.gov/healthinformation/
bipolarmenu.cfm

This area of the NIMH Web site features basic information about bipolar comorbidity disorder as well as related information on comorbidity, medications, and suicide risk. In addition, the site provides information on current clinical trials.

International Society for Bipolar Disorders
www.isbd.org

This non-profit organization promotes awareness of bipolar disorder in society at large and among mental health professionals, fostering research on all aspects of the illness and promoting international collaboration on research and development of improved treatment options. The Web site features updates from the Stanley Medication Research Institute (SMRI) treatment trials as well as information on ongoing studies at the Western Psychiatric Institute and Clinic on bipolar disorder and youth.

Mood Disorders Society of Canada
www.mooddisorderscanada.ca

This site features a variety of resources including copies of Canadian mental health policy reports and useful links to international Web sites dealing with mood disorders.

American Foundation for Suicide Prevention (AFSP)
www.afsp.org

Dedicated to preventing suicide, this organization is involved in educational and advocacy programs as well as support services for those impacted by suicide. The AFSP Web site lists educational resources, and provides information about grants, suicide prevention programs, and advocacy/public policy efforts.

Harvard Bipolar Research Program
www.manicdepressive.org

This site is sponsored by the Massachusetts General Hospital Bipolar Clinic and Research Program (formerly Harvard Bipolar Research Program) and is devoted to educating physicians and patients as well as the greater community about bipolar disorder. The Web site's "Tools for Clinicians" area provides downloadable copies of the Clinical Monitoring Form (CMF), Affective Disorders Evaluation (ADE), and Clinical Self-Report Form for

INTRODUCTION

PRESENTATION

CLINICAL PROCESS

PHARMACOTHERAPY

RESOURCES

clinician use as well as helpful information and samples of mood charts and treatment contracts.

Emory University Women's Mental Health Program
www.emorywomensprogram.org

This program, established in 1991, focuses on assessment and treatment of emotional disorders during pregnancy and the postpartum period. The Web site offers information on the clinical program, research programs, and intake packet used as well as a wealth of links and articles on related topics.

Massachusetts General Hospital – Center for Women's Mental Health
www.womensmentalhealth.org

The Center is dedicated to evaluating and treating psychiatric disorders associated with female reproductive function. In addition to an area specifically devoted to patient information on the Web site, there is information about the Center's clinical program and research studies as well as discussions of "hot topics," new research at the center, and extensive Web links.

Glossary

A

abnormal grief — acute grief persisting beyond the typical two to four months that may contribute to depressive symptoms or exacerbate a bipolar depressive episode

absolute starting dose — amount of medication given when the patient first takes it

active listening — a way of listening that focuses entirely on what the other person is saying and confirms understanding of both the message content and the emotions and feelings underlying the message to ensure accurate understanding

add-on treatment — the addition of a new medication to already ongoing treatment

affect — the visible expression of subjectively experienced emotion

akathisia — a state of motor restlessness, ranging from a feeling of inner disquiet to an inability to sit still or lie quietly

algorithms — an organized, often specific set of recommendations that are evidence-based, often informed by expert consensus opinion when there are inadequate studies to inform treatment decisions

amygdala — a collection of subcortical nuclei that are part of the limbic system and involved in phasic regulation of emotion, particularly arousal

anhedonia — inability to gain pleasure from normally pleasurable experiences

assertive communication techniques — the systematic procedure that helps patients honestly express opinions, feelings, attitudes, and rights (without undue anxiety) in a way that doesn't infringe on the rights of others

attributional style — one's tendencies in making causal explanations about a variety of intra- and interpersonal events in their lives

atypical antipsychotics — the class of antipsychotic medications with (overall) less extra-pyramidal side-effects

atypical features — mood reactivity and at least two of the following: increased appetite or weight gain, excessive sleep, the sensation that one's limbs are too heavy to move, and a long-standing pattern of sensitivity to perceived interpersonal rejection

B

behavioral rehearsal — rehearsing new responses to problematic situations

C

catatonic features — clinical features characterized by marked psychomotor disturbance that may involve immobility, excessive motor activity, extreme negativism, inability or refusal to speak, peculiar voluntary movements or speech

circadian rhythms — the daily regulation of sleep-wake cycles and activity-to-activity patterns

cotransmitters — two molecules released from the same synapse that act on an adjacent neuron, both of which are physiologically active

crossover design — a type of clinical study where patients are randomized to one treatment arm, then at some point during the study will be "crossed over" to receive the other treatment option

D

delusions — false, fixed, odd, or unusual beliefs about external reality that are not accepted by other members of the person's culture or subculture, yet are firmly sustained despite clear evidence to the contrary

depression — a mood state characterized by sadness or irritability, and/or lack of interest in previously enjoyed activities; associated with other symptoms, such as irritability, sleep disturbance, inappropriate guilt, cognitive dysfunction, and thoughts of death or suicide

derailment — quality of speech characterized by loose associations or an inability to stay on topic; problematic connection between ideas

dopamine — a neurotransmitter in the central nervous system that affects the synthesis of epinephrine

dysphoric hypomania — a mood state characterized by abnormally and persistently irritable mood, increased energy, and symptoms of depression that do not meet full criteria for a major depressive episode

E

epileptic seizure — an uncontrolled discharge of brain cells that spread throughout the brain, causing seizures with associated brief loss of consciousness and bladder control or aberrant excitable neural activity that stays localized (e.g., isolated limb movements, temporary blindness)

episode — symptoms of mania, hypomania, and/or depression meeting DSM-IV criteria

euthymia — normal range of mood with no evidence of mania, hypomania, or depression

evidence-based studies — medication information gained through placebo-controlled, double-blind studies (where neither the patient nor physician know who receives the "active" pill with medication versus the "sugar" pill)

executive functions — those functions of the brain carried out by the prefrontal and frontal cortex: managing stimuli, marshaling appropriate responses, and modulating impulses, which are all disrupted in manic states and major depression

expressed emotion — a qualitative expression of the amount of emotion displayed in family or group settings, often involving hostility, critical attitudes, and emotionality that may adversely impact recovery and relapse of mood disorders

F

flight of ideas — rapid change of topics, loosely linked together

fMRI (functional MRI) — an imaging technique that uses the magnetic properties of blood to map brain functioning

G

genetic-laden — families that have multiple members with impairing mood disorders

goal-directed behavior — behavior directed towards accomplishing a specific task(s)

grandiosity — exaggerated belief or claims of one's importance, identity, or capacity; when of psychotic proportions, manifested as delusions of great wealth, power, or fame

H

habitus — body build, can refer to weight impact of medications

hallucinations — sensory perceptions (seeing, hearing, feeling, and smelling) in the absence of an outside stimulus

hippocampus — an important part of the limbic system involved in working memory and other functions

hormone receptors — a group of molecules that have diverse function throughout the brain and the body (e.g., steroid or estrogen receptors)

hyperphagia — abnormally increased appetite for and consumption of food, thought to be associated with a lesion or injury in the hypothalamus

hypersomnia — a condition in which one sleeps for an excessively long time but is normal in the waking intervals

hypomania — a mood state characterized by increased energy, excitement, irritable mood, and usually mild, decreased sleep that do not meet the diagnostic criteria for a full manic episode

I

iatrogenic — induced in a patient by a physician's activity, manner, or therapy

impulsivity — taking action with limited thought to consequences

insight — understanding or awareness of one's mental or emotional condition

interitem reliability — degree to which scores on individual items agree with each other; an estimate of the extent to which the instrument is measuring a single construct

interrater reliability — degree that different raters agree on answers to questions on a given instrument for either diagnosis or clinical symptoms

M

maintenance treatment — an ongoing treatment believed to prevent or minimize the development of new manic, hypomanic, depressive, or mixed episodes

major neurochemical receptor groups — neurotransmitter substances believed important in normal and abnormal brain functioning

mania — a severely impairing mood state characterized by an elevated or irritable mood, decreased sleep, high energy, impulsive behavior, and increased goal-directed behavior causing significant disruption in a person's life

melancholic features — loss of interest or pleasure in all, or almost all activities, and lack of reactivity to usually pleasurable stimuli

mixed episodes — periods during which symptoms of a manic and a depressive episode (that meet DSM-IV criteria) are present at the same time

mixed states — periods during which symptoms of a hypomania and a sub-syndromal depression (that do not meet DSM-IV criteria) are present at the same time

MRI (Magnetic Resonance Imaging) — a technique using magnetic fields and radio waves to produce images of brain structures

N

neuropeptides — brain chemicals or medications that either decrease cell death and/or increase the birth of new brain cells (i.e., neurogenesis)

neuroprotective effect — the function of neuropeptides to either decrease cell death and/or increase neurogenesis

neurotransmitter — a chemical in the brain that transmits information between the nerve cells

neurotrophins — a class of molecules, which trigger changes in the second messenger system(s), thereby increasing cell survival and new cell growth

P

paranormal phenomena — altered perceptions experienced by the patient but not those around them, [e.g., hearing voices (auditory hallucinations), smelling burning rubber (olfactory hallucinations), etc.] as well as déjà vu, the sense of having already experienced what is now happening

PET imaging — technology that uses positron-labeled molecules and an oxygen blood flow tracer to develop images of brain activity

pleomorphic — occurring in many different distinct forms

prodromal — precursor to a full episode, or less than criteria for a full-blown episode; sub-syndromal symptoms

psychoeducational package — a treatment approach that includes multiple methods for educating the patient, such as: written, visual, and interactive materials to facilitate education about the disorder and treatment

psychosis —extreme impairment of a person's ability to think clearly, perceive things accurately, respond emotionally, communicate effectively, understand reality, and behave appropriately

R

rapid cycling — four or more manic, hypomanic, or depressive episodes in any 12-month period

rate of initial titration — the rate by which a medication is increased to what is believed to be a minimum effective dose

role-playing — helping a person acquire new communication skills by having them act out conversations

S

seasonal pattern — onset and remission of mood episodes occurring at characteristic times of the year

sensitivity — the degree to which the instrument correctly identifies patients that do have the disorder

serotonin — a neurotransmitter from the indoleamine group that affects central nervous system functioning

somatization — multiple physical complaints involving any body system

specificity — the degree to which the instrument correctly identifies patients that do not have the disorder

specifiers — DSM-IV-defined categories for specific symptoms that may occur with bipolar disorder, such as psychotic or atypical symptoms

SPECT imaging — a single photon emission where image intensity is directly correlated to cerebral perfusion or blood flow to develop images of brain activity

sub-syndromal — symptoms of mania, hypomania, or depression not meeting episode criteria

T

T-scores — standardized scores based on 0 to 100, with 50 as a mean

tangentiality — speech characterized by giving unrelated answers to direct questions and frequently changing topics

tardive dyskinesia — a neurological syndrome characterized by repetitive, involuntary, purposeless movements

temporal lobe — a large lobe of each cerebral hemisphere that is in front of the occipital lobe and is believed to be involved in memory, mood regulation, and impulsivity

transcranial magnetic stimulation (rTMS) — a therapeutic technique using a magnetic force to stimulate neurons in the brain

V

vagal nerve stimulation — an FDA-approved treatment for refractory epilepsy and depression now being explored for bipolar disorder

Index

Trisha Suppes, M.D., Ph.D.
Statement of Disclosure

Sources of Funding for Clinical Grants: Dr. Suppes is a principal or co-investigator on research studies sponsored by Abbott Laboratories, Astra Zeneca, GlaxoSmith Kline Pharmaceuticals, JDS Pharmaceuticals, Janssen Pharmaceutica, National Institutes of Mental Health, Novartis Pharmaceuticals, Pfizer Inc., The Stanley Medical Research Institute, and Wyeth Pharmaceuticals Inc.

Consulting Agreements/Advisory Boards: Dr. Suppes is a consultant to, or member of the scientific advisory boards of Abbott Laboratories, Astra Zeneca, Bristol Myers Squibb, Eli Lilly Research Laboratories, GlaxoSmithKline Pharmaceuticals, JDS Pharmaceuticals, Janssen Pharmaceutica, Novartis Pharmaceutical, Ortho McNeil Pharmaceutical, Pfizer Inc., Shire Pharmaceutical, Solvay, and UCB Pharma.

Speaking Bureaus: Dr. Suppes serves on speaking bureaus for Astra Zeneca and Glaxo Smith Kline Pharmaceuticals.

J. Sloan Manning, M.D.
Statement of Disclosure

I am a consultant to and on the speaker's bureau of Eli Lilly and AstraZeneca.

Paul E. Keck, Jr. M.D.
Statement of Disclosure

Research Grants: Dr. Keck is a principal or co-investigator on research studies sponsored by Abbott Laboratories, the American Diabetes Association, AstraZeneca, Bristol-Myers Squibb, GlaxoSmithKline, Elan, Eli Lilly, Janssen Pharmaceutica, Merck, National Institute of Mental Health (NIMH), National Institute of Drug Abuse (NIDA), Organon, Ortho-McNeil, Pfizer, the Stanley Medical Research Institute (SMRI), and UCB Pharma.

Consultant/Scientific Advisory Boards: Dr. Keck is a consultant to, or member of the scientific advisory boards of Abbott Laboratories, AstraZeneca Pharmaceuticals, Bristol-Myers Squibb, GlaxoSmithKline, Janssen Pharmaceutica, Jazz Pharmaceuticals, Eli Lilly and Company, Novartis, Ortho-McNeil, Pfizer, UCB Pharma, Shire, and Wyeth.

Compact Clinicals' Publications

For Physicians

Bipolar Disorder: Treatment and Management
By Trisha Suppes, MD, PhD and Paul E. Keck, Jr., MD

Decoding Bipolar Disorder: Practical Treatment and Management
By Trisha Suppes, MD, PhD, J. Sloan Manning, MD, and Paul E. Keck, Jr., MD

For Clinicians

Attention Deficit Hyperactivity Disorder
The Latest Assessment and Treatment Strategies
By C. Keith Conners, PhD

Bipolar Disorder
The Latest Assessment and Treatment Strategies
By Trisha Suppes MD, PhD and Ellen B. Dennehy, PhD

Borderline Personality Disorder
The Latest Assessment and Treatment Strategies
By Melanie Dean, PhD

Conduct Disorders
The Latest Assessment and Treatment Strategies
By J. Mark Eddy, PhD

Depression in Adults
The Latest Assessment and Treatment Strategies
By Anton Tolman, PhD

Obsessive Compulsive Disorder
The Latest Assessment and Treatment Strategies
By Gail Steketee, PhD and Teresa Pigott, MD

Post-Traumatic and Acute Stress Disorders
The Latest Assessment and Treatment Strategies
By Matthew J. Friedman, MD, PhD

For more information or to order, contact:
Compact Clinicals
7205 N.W. Waukomis Drive
Kansas City, MO 64151
1-800-408-8830